Recent Results in Cancer Research 120

Recent Results in Cancer Research

Volume 110
P. Schlag, P. Hohenberger, U. Metzger (Eds.):
Combined Modality Therapy of Gastrointestinal Tract Cancer
1988. 105 figures, 122 tables. XVII, 301. ISBN 3-540-18610-7

Volume 111
H. Scheurlen, R. Kay, M. Baum (Eds.):
Cancer Clinical Trials: A Critical Appraisal
1988. 37 figures, 53 tables. IX, 272. ISBN 3-540-19098-8

Volume 112
L. Schmid, H.-J. Senn (Eds.): AIDS-Related Neoplasias
1988. 23 figures, 35 tables. IX, 97. ISBN 3-540-19227-1

Volume 113
U. Eppenberger, A. Goldhirsch (Eds.):
Endocrine Therapy and Growth Regulation of Breast Cancer
1989. 26 figures, 17 tables. IX, 92. ISBN 3-540-50456-7

Volume 114
P. Boyle, C.S. Muir, E. Grundmann (Eds.): Cancer Mapping
1989. 97 figures, 64 tables. IX, 277. ISBN 3-540-50490-7

Volume 115
H.-J. Senn, A. Goldhirsch, R.D. Gelber, B. Osterwalder (Eds.):
Adjuvant Therapy of Primary Breast Cancer
1989. 64 figures, 94 tables. XVI, 296. ISBN 3-540-18810-X

Volume 116
K.W. Brunner, H. Fleisch, H.-J. Senn (Eds.):
Bisphosphonates and Tumor Osteolysis
1989. 22 figures, 6 tables. IX, 78. ISBN 3-540-50560-1

Volume 117
V. Diehl, M. Pfreundschuh, M. Loeffler (Eds.):
New Aspects in the Diagnosis and Treatment of Hodgkin's Disease
1989. 71 figures, 91 tables. XIV, 283. ISBN 3-540-51124-5

Volume 118
L. Beck, E. Grundmann, R. Ackermann, H.-D. Röher (Eds.):
Hormone-Related Malignant Tumors
1990. 83 figures, 91 tables. XI, 269. ISBN 3-540-51258-6

Volume 119
S. Brünner, B. Langfeldt (Eds.):
Advances in Breast Cancer Detection
1990. 53 figures, 51 tables. X1, 195. ISBN 3-540-52089-9

Pierre Band (Ed.)

Occupational Cancer Epidemiology

With 23 Figures and 59 Tables

Springer-Verlag Berlin Heidelberg New York
London Paris Tokyo Hong Kong Barcelona

Pierre Band, M.D.
Head, Division of Epidemiology
Biometry & Occupational Oncology
Cancer Control Agency of British Columbia
600 West 10th Avenue
Vancouver, B.C. V5Z 4E6, Canada

ISBN-13:978-3-642-84070-8 e-ISBN-13:978-3-642-84068-5
DOI: 10.1007/978-3-642-84068-5

Library of Congress Cataloging-in-Publication Data
Occupational cancer epidemiology/Pierre Band (ed.).
p.cm. — (Recent results in cancer research; 120)
ISBN-13:978-3-642-84070-8 (U.S.: alk. paper)
1. Cancer-Etiology. 2. Cancer-Risk factors. 3. Occupational diseases.
4. Cancer-Epidemiology. I. Band, P.R. (Pierre R.), 1935- . II. Series.
[DNLM: 1. Neoplasms—epidemiology. 2. Occupational Diseases—
epidemiology. W1 RE106P v. 120/QZ 200 015]
RC261.R35 vol. 120 [RC268.48] 616.99'4 s-dc20
[614.5'999] DNLM/DLC 90-9570

Softcover reprint of the hardcover 1st edition 1990

Typesetting: Macmillan India Ltd., Bangalore-25, India

2125/3140-543210-Printed on acid-free paper.

Preface

The identification of occupational cancer risk factors and of carcinogens in the workplace is assuming increasing importance in cancer epidemiology. This book, which contains the proceedings of a symposium held in Vancouver in June 1988, combines overviews by experts on substantive topics and methodologic issues of broad interest in occupational cancer epidemiology. Among the former are state of the art reviews emphasizing recent data and new and innovative analytic approaches. The substantive topics include discussion of cancer risks from exposure to complex organic mixtures, asbestos and man-made fibers, herbicides, radon, and electromagnetic fields. Risk assessment, exposure assessment, and analysis of occupational cohort studies are examples of the methodologic issues addressed. This book provides basic information and opens perspectives on new areas of research.

In organizing our symposium we were greatly assisted by Betty Fata and Kim Rust of Venue West Conference Ltd. We appreciate the financial support received from the following:

Cancer Control Agency of British Columbia
Alcan Aluminium Ltd.
National Health Research & Development Program
Workers' Compensation Board of British Columbia
Purdue Frederick Inc.
Rhone-Poulenc Pharma Inc.
London Drugs Ltd.
Ciba-Geigy Canada Ltd.
Bristol-Myers Pharmaceutical Group
Schering Canada Inc.
Hoffmann-La Roche Ltd.
Sterling Drug Ltd.
Parke-Davis Canada Inc.
Beecham Laboratories
Pfizer Canada Inc.
Roussel Canada Inc.
Novopharm

Contents

*List of Contributors**

---

* The address of the principal author is given on the first page of each contribution.

[1] Page on which contribution begins.

Role of Epidemiology in Health Risk Assessment

D. Krewski[1], D. Wigle[1], D.B. Clayson[1], and G.R. Howe[2]*

[1] Health Protection Branch, Health and Welfare Canada, Ottawa, Ontario K1A 0L2, Canada
[2] National Cancer Institute of Canada, University of Toronto, Toronto, Ontario, M5S I18, Canada

Introduction

The process of health risk assessment has been the subject of systematic study in recent years. For example, interdisciplinary groups established by the U.S. National Research Council (NRC 1983) and the World Health Organization (WHO 1985) have developed models for risk assessment and risk management. These investigations have provided clear frameworks within which questions pertaining to health risks may be addressed. This has proven useful in distinguishing between the scientific and extrascientific dimensions of risk assessment, and in ensuring that all relevant factors are given proper attention in risk management decisions.

Most of our information on environmental and occupational health risks is based on epidemiological investigation of people exposed to the risk factor of interest or on toxicological experiments conducted on nonhuman test systems.

Although epidemiological studies have the advantage of providing information directly on humans, they are subject to certain limitations. Epidemiological studies are only possible after human exposure has occurred, and after the health effect of interest has had sufficient time to develop. With chronic diseases such as cancer, this induction period may span one or two generations. There may also be technical problems in exposure assessment and adjustment for the presence of confounding risk factors in observational studies of human populations.

In contrast, toxicological studies afford the opportunity to determine possible adverse effects before human exposure is permitted. Similarly, because experiments are conducted in a carefully controlled laboratory environment, the toxicologist can attain a degree of precision denied to the epidemiologist who must work with a heterogeneous human population exposed to a wide variety of risk factors influencing health status. However, because toxicological studies are conducted in nonhuman test systems, this precision is achieved under penalty of

---

* The authors would like to thank Terry Chernis for bibliographic assistance in preparing this article.

Recent Results in Cancer Research, Vol. 120

introducing the need for uncertain extrapolations from the test system employed to humans.

In this paper, we examine the complementary roles of epidemiology and toxicology in human health risk assessment. We begin with a description of a model for risk assessment and risk management which will serve to place the role of epidemiology in health risk assessment in perspective. We then provide a brief description of the different epidemiological protocols which have been used in health risk assessment. Case studies of active and passive smoking as well as saccharin and formaldehyde are presented to illustrate the complementary roles of epidemiology and toxicology in health risk assessment. The resolution of discrepancies between epidemiological and toxicological findings is treated next, including the use of weight of evidence approaches for combining information from both sources to arrive at an overall assessment of risk. Finally, we present a summary of our main findings.

Risk Assessment and Risk Management

A number of recent studies have examined the process of health risk assessment and risk management. For example, several national and international organizations have proposed specific models to describe this process (see Krewski and Birkwood 1987, for a recent detailed review). These models exhibit many similarities and serve to clarify the important elements of risk assessment and risk management, including the role of epidemiology in this process (Krewski 1987).

Building on these foundations, a Working Group on Risk Assessment and Risk Management (1988) developed a model for use within the Environmental Health Directorate of Health and Welfare Canada (Fig. 1). The first two steps involve the identification of a specific environmental hazard and the estimation of the corresponding levels of risk. These two steps combined involve the analysis of epidemiological and toxicological data, and together comprise what may be termed risk analysis.

Following risk analysis, the risk manager may consider a variety of options for the protection of human health. These risk management strategies may be broadly classified as regulatory, economic, advisory or technological (Krewski and Birkwood 1988). While direct regulation continues to be widely used, nonregulatory alternatives have received increasing attention in recent years. For example, economic options rely on economic incentives and disincentives to reduce environmental pollution. Advisory approaches rely on the provision of advice to promote risk avoidance. Formal regulations may also be avoided if new technological developments are used for pollution abatement. These options are not mutually exclusive, as demonstrated by the use of a combination of all four approaches in attempting to control acidic deposition in Canada (Burnett et al. 1988).

The selection of a suitable risk management strategy is complex, and is frequently charged with social and political overtones (Somers 1983, 1984). As

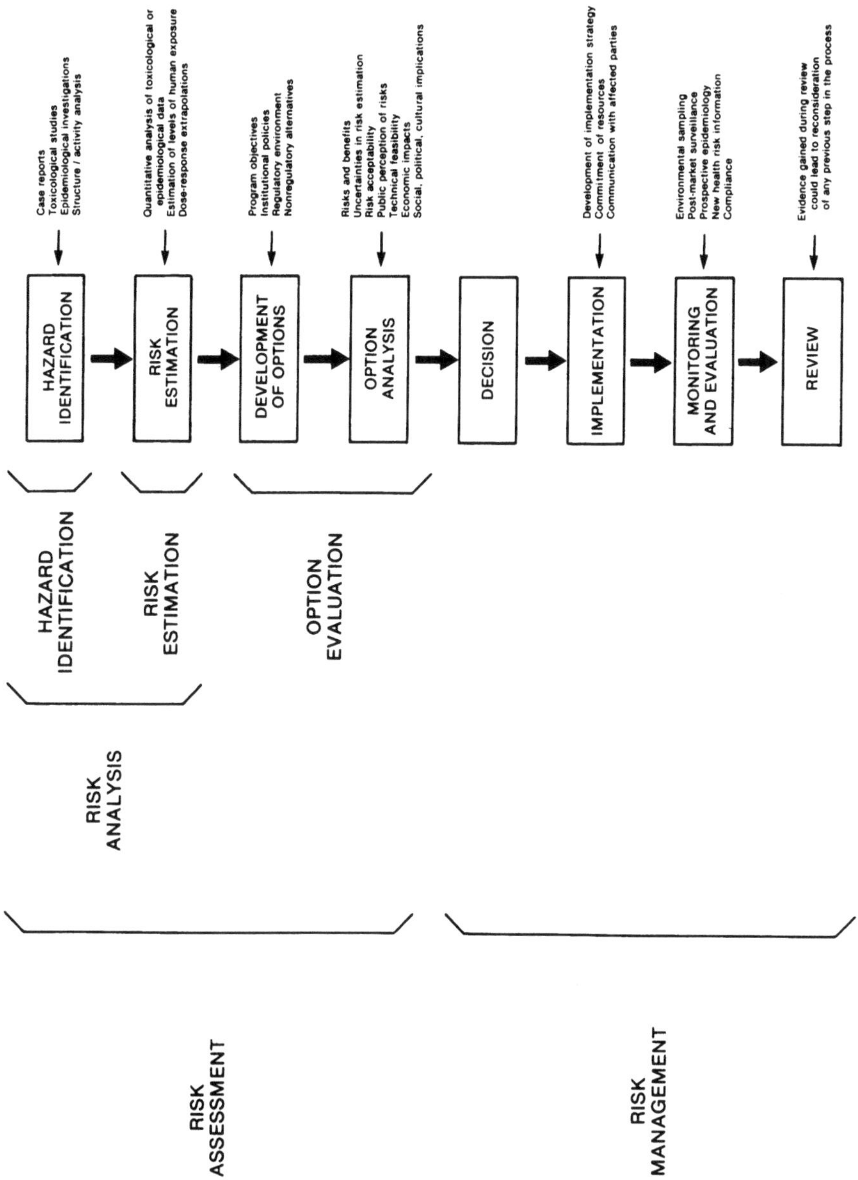

Fig. 1. A model for risk assessment and risk management

an aid to decision making, it may be helpful to apply formal program evaluation techniques to assess effects on human health, the environment and social structure, and the economic consequences that flow from them (Torrance and Krewski 1985). Although such analyses are not intended to generate a clear-cut decision, they are of value in objectively evaluating all of the available data, and summarizing the results in a form that will assist in arriving at a solution to the problem at hand (Krewski et al. 1989b).

Public perception of risk is an important consideration in risk assessment (Krewski et al. 1987). In contrast to risk analysis, risk perception is a subjective process by which individuals intuitively assess risk. Because of human limitations in information processing, the public often misjudges risk and adopts views which may be at odds with objectively derived estimates. Decision makers need to be aware of public perception of the risk associated with different hazards, and give these views proper consideration in selecting an appropriate risk management strategy.

Communication of risk related information is clearly a critical part of risk management (Covello et al. 1987; Davies et al. 1987). It is important that risk data be expressed in understandable terms, and that effective channels of communication be established among individuals and institutions involved in the assessment of risk. Examination of models of risk communication has provided some insight into the risk communication processes. For example, the communications processes model proposed by Leiss and Krewski (1989) is based on the notion that risk communication is defined by the interplay of two domains, called the expert sphere and the public sphere. This model highlights the tension between technically assessed and perceived risk, which is considered a distinctive feature of risk communication. Epidemiology can play a major role in risk communication through the transmission of information on health risks from the expert sphere to the public sphere in a manner which can be appreciated by the population at large.

Epidemiological Studies

The health problems of people in developed countries are generally well documented, particularly serious conditions such as cancer and heart disease. Descriptive epidemiological studies can provide useful statistical measures of the health impact of such diseases. As indicated in Fig. 2, cancer is by far the most serious disease facing the Canadian population when ranked by potential years of life lost (D.T. Wigle and Y. Mao, Health and Welfare Canada, Ottawa, unpublished data). Epidemiological information of this type is of use in establishing new directions for measuring health status and in setting public health priorities (Glass 1986).

Ecologic epidemiological studies involve comparisons of population exposure with the occurrence of a particular disease over time or across geographic areas. For example, consider the longitudinal data on tobacco consumption in Canada and lung cancer incidence shown in Fig. 3 (Wigle et al. 1986). Allowing

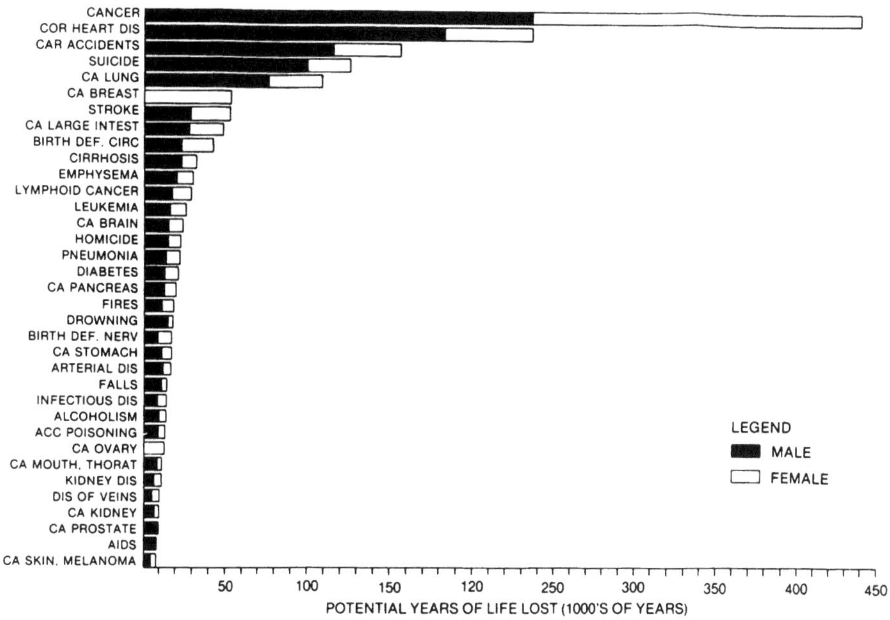

Fig. 2. Major health problems ranked by potential year of life lost

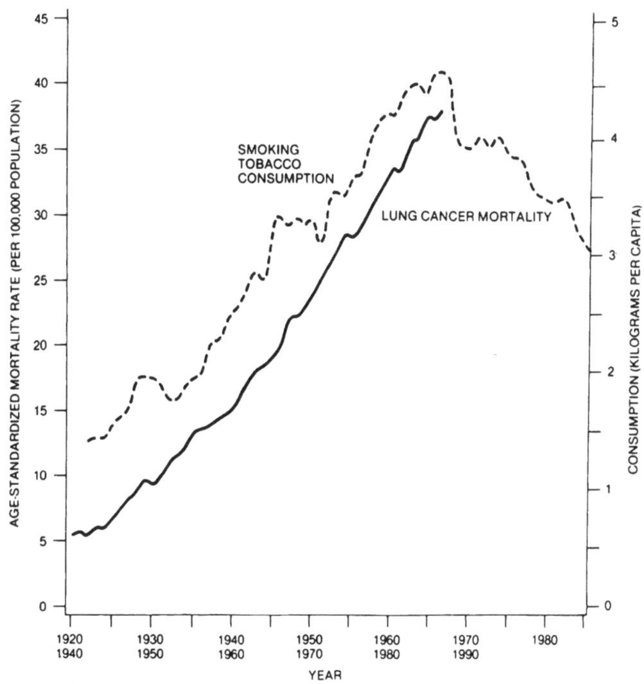

Fig. 3. Smoking tobacco consumption (1920–1985) and age standardized lung cancer mortality rates (1940–1986)

for a 20-year time lag, these results reveal a strong association between tobacco consumption and lung cancer. The problem with such studies is the difficulty in concluding that a causal relationship exists, as illustrated by a similarly strong association in Fig. 4 between the number of pairs of brooding storks and the human birth rate in the Federal Republic of Germany (Sies 1988). As will become clear further on, these latter data are not presented as contraindicating the well-established adverse health effects of tobacco consumption. Rather, they are included to emphasize the need for a careful comprehensive evaluation of epidemiologic data in assessing causality (Hoel and Landrigan 1987). For example, determinations of causality should include consideration of criteria such as the strength and consistency of the association, the temporal relationship between cause and effect, the biological gradient and specificity of the association, and the biological possibility of the association in light of known information on disease etiology (Hill 1965).

Because of limitations such as those discussed above, ecologic studies serve primarily to suggest the need for a more rigorous epidemiological investigation. In case-control studies, information on the etiology of the disease under study is obtained retrospectively on both affected and unaffected individuals (Breslow and Day 1980). The sampling of diseased subjects coupled with a scheme for collecting exposure information retrospectively makes this design well suited to testing etiologic hypotheses for specific rare diseases. Unfortunately, information on exposures such as prescription drug usage and certain lifestyle habits such as diet is often less than adequate, especially when it is necessary to look as far into the past as with cancer. Nonetheless, retrospective epidemiological studies have been able to identify certain hazards, such as vaginal cancer in young women whose mothers were given the synthetic hormone diethylstilbestrol for pregnancy maintenance (Herbst et al. 1975).

In cohort studies, information on exposure and possible confounding factors is obtained for comparison with an unexposed reference group (Breslow and

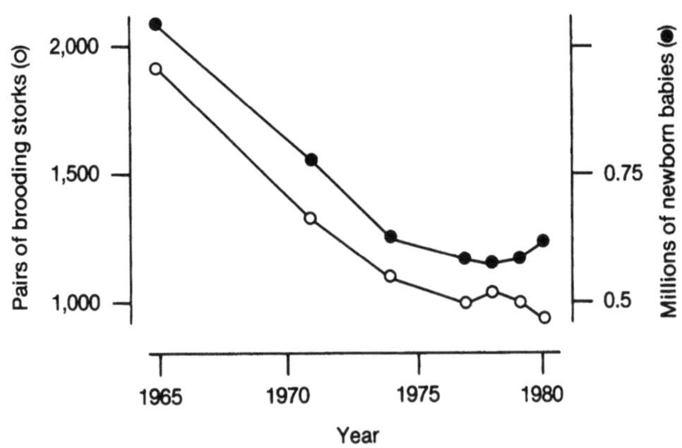

Fig. 4. Human birthrate and stork brooding in Federal Republic of Germany (1965–1980)

Day 1987). The population is then monitored over a period of time, with the follow-up period depending on the cohort size, the background incidence rate of the disease or diseases of interest, and the desired relative risk detection limit. Historical exposure records such as those on occupational exposure histories may be used to reduce the time required to accumulate adequate person-years of observation. The direct sampling of subjects with variable exposures coupled with a plan of recording health effects as they occur is appropriate for relatively common diseases such as coronary heart disease, motor vehicle injury, common infections or general mortality. Cohort studies will require large sample sizes for the study of rare diseases and may require extended follow-up time in studies of chronic diseases such as cancer. Nonetheless, cohort studies have demonstrated a doubling in overall mortality due to smoking (Doll and Peto 1976).

Administrative records offer the potential means to conduct low-cost large-scale epidemiological investigations without the need to collect new data. Much valuable information on the health status of the Canadian population is collected on an ongoing basis in the form of hospital records, health insurance data, disease registries and national statistics on morbidity and mortality. The use of existing computerized databases for epidemiological purposes often requires that linkages be made between records on the same individual that may reside in several different files. The record linkage technology originally proposed by Newcombe (1967) has evolved over the years to the point where it has been successfully applied in a number of major studies such as that conducted by Howe et al. (1979) on the effects of isoniazid on tuberculosis patients. Studies of this type are currently underway within the Health Protection Branch to investigate possible relationships between cancer mortality and occupational exposure to radiation and certain agricultural chemicals.

Because of ethical problems, randomized study designs for toxic effects in humans are not feasible. However, many randomized trials of risk factor interventions have been conducted to assess the effectiveness of drugs, surgical procedures, behavioural changes and dietary changes. For example, a randomized trial for treatment of stable angina revealed virtually identical 11-year survival rates for persons treated with coronary artery bypass surgery and those treated medically (Veterans Administration Coronary Artery Bypass Surgery Cooperative Study Group 1984). Recently, the feasibility of a trial to determine the effect of reducing dietary fat content on the risk of breast cancer among middle-aged women has been assessed in the United States. The results of this study are not yet available.

In sum, epidemiological studies have provided considerable information on the environmental determinants of cancer in humans (Schottenfeld and Fraumeni 1982; Magnus 1982). These data have recently been used by Doll and Peto (1981) and Miller (1984) to estimate the fraction of total cancer mortality attributable to specific causes (Table 1). Although these figures involve some judgment on the part of these investigators, there is good evidence that tobacco is responsible for about 30% of the total cancer burden. Estimates of the proportion of cancer mortality attributable to diet were similar, although

Table 1. Estimates of the percentage of cancer deaths attributable to known causal factors

Factors	Canada (Miller 1984)	United States (Doll and Peto 1981)
Tobacco	26	30
Diet	32	35
Occupation	9	4
Radiation[a]	2	3
Alcohol	6	3
Reproductive patterns	4	7
Sexual activity	3	
Licit drugs	1	1
Viruses	?	5
General environment	?	2

[a] Including sunlight.

subject to much greater uncertainty. The remaining determinants of cancer were all considered to have attributable risks of less than 10%.

Applications

The role of epidemiological data in health risk assessment may be further illustrated using a series of practical applications. The four case studies presented here were selected to reflect the different ways in which epidemiology can contribute to human health risk assessment, depending on the magnitude and nature of the health effect involved and on the strength of the available data. These examples were also selected to contrast the complementary roles of epidemiology and toxicology in risk assessment.

Active Smoking

Cigarette smoking is one of the most important environmental factors contributing to premature cancer mortality in North America (Wigle 1984). There are approximately 3800 identified components in cigarette tobacco (DHHS 1980, 1982). Several of the components in the gaseous and particulate phases of cigarette smoke are mutagenic or carcinogenic. Smoking directly exposes tissues in the oral cavity, throat, larynx, trachea, bronchis, lung and esophagus to these substances. Soluble substances in smoke are absorbed into the bloodstream and can exert their toxic effects on every responsive system of the body.

The fact that cigarette smoking presaged a major health disaster did not become apparent until Wynder and Graham made their first epidemiological survey of cigarette smoking and lung cancer in 1950 (see Wigle 1985, for a historical review). Epidemiological evidence on the consequences of cigarette smoking thereafter accumulated rapidly, with retrospective and prospective studies demonstrating that the risk for cancer of the lung, larynx, oral cavity, esophagus, pancreas, kidney and bladder is increased among cigarette smokers as opposed to nonsmokers (Wigle et al. 1980; Wynder and Hoffman 1982; Wigle 1984).

Canada's male lung cancer mortality rate increased sharply from 1930, corresponding to a rapid growth in the number of smokers during and after World War I (Mao and Smith 1983). Canada's female lung cancer mortality rate increased in a similar manner to that of males, but with a 25-year time lag (Mao et al. 1982). If this trend continues, more Canadian woman will die from lung cancer than breast cancer by 1990 (Wigle et al. 1986), the latter being the current leading cause of cancer death for women.

Cigarette smoking is not only responsible for many smoking-related diseases, but may also modify the effects of other risk factors (Saraci 1987). The interaction of smoking and other risk factors may be seen synergistic as with the lung cancer risk among workers exposed to asbestos (Selikoff and Hammond 1975) or radon (NRC 1988). Synergistic effects between alcohol consumption and cigarette smoking with respect to the development of the cancer of mouth and pharynx may also occur (Rothman and Keller 1972; NRC 1988).

Toxicology has, for a number of reasons, made a relatively minor contribution to the development of our knowledge on the health effects of cigarette smoking. First, the presence of a large exposed human population has made the use of surrogate species unnecessary for the identification of the hazard. Second, at the time of rapid development of interest in the health consequences of cigarette smoking, knowledge of the techniques of inhalation toxicology was only poorly developed. Third, surrogate species appeared relatively insensitive to the chronic adverse effects of cigarette smoking possibly because the acute toxicity of tobacco smoke precluded the dose exaggeration that has proved so useful in investigating single chemicals. Laboratory studies have therefore concentrated on attempts to quantify the adverse consequences of smoke from modified cigarettes developed to determine whether it is possible to develop a safer product (Gori 1976).

The experimental techniques used for the study of the adverse effects of tobacco smoking include machine smoking of cigarettes, the collection of the main-stream smoke in liquid nitrogen cooled traps and the induction of mouse skin tumors by painting this condensate, or fractions thereof, onto mouse skin. Such studies have shown that tobacco-smoke condensates, as well as those from the combination of other organic materials, are carcinogenic. This work has rendered the hypothesis that it might be possible to devise a safer cigarette highly questionable. In addition, a host of different chemical carcinogens have been identified as being present in small amounts in tobacco-smoke concentrate. Thus, this condensate contains traces of the human bladder carcinogen, 2-naphthylamine, as well as other aromatic amines (Hoffman et al. 1969), and a number of tobacco-specific N-nitrosamines capable of inducing cancer in several tissues in experimental animals (Hoffman et al. 1980).

Collishaw et al. (1988) provided estimates of the number of deaths in Canada due to active smoking. The number of deaths N_s due to smoking is given by

$$N_s = N \times PAR,$$

where N is the annual number of deaths in Canada and PAR is the population attributable risk for mortality for those who have ever been smokers. The number of deaths by age and sex is available directly from the Mortality Data Base maintained by Statistics Canada. The PAR is estimated from epidemiologic studies using the relationship

$$PAR = p(RR\text{-}1)/\{p(RR\text{-}1) + 1\},$$

where RR is the relative risk for those who have ever been smokers and p is the proportion of the population who have ever been smokers. Collishaw et al. (1988) used data from the 1985 General Social Survey conducted by Statistics Canada to estimate p along with data from Godley (1974) on a sample of 20 000 death records in the United States to estimate the RR by age and sex. This analysis suggests that about 35 000 deaths in Canada may be attributable to ever smoking. Johansen et al. (1987) obtained a similar estimate based on estimates of p and RR derived from a follow-up mortality study of individuals from the Nutrition Canada Survey conducted in 1972.

Passive Smoking

Lung cancer is the leading cause of cancer deaths in males in Canada, and is the second leading cause among females. In 1988, there will be an estimated 9300 deaths from lung cancer among males and 4100 deaths among females (G.B. Hill et al. 1988). As discussed previously, the causal nature of the association between active smoking and lung cancer is well established (IARC 1986), with a very large proportion of lung cancer accounted for by active smoking.

In view of the large number of deaths from lung cancer that occur in Canada, there remains a substantial number of such deaths which are not attributable to active smoking. It is thus of interest to determine to what extent the cancer burden unexplained by active smoking may be attributed to passive smoking. Passive smokers are exposed at lower levels to the constituents of tobacco smoke than are active smokers, with the possible exception that chemically unstable consituents may have largely decomposed before the passive smoker inhales sidestream smoke.

The first studies to indicate a possible increased risk of lung cancer from passive smoking came from Japan and Greece, countries with a larger proportion of female nonsmokers than North America. On the basis of a large cohort study, Hirayama (1981) reported a RR of 1.8 for female nonsmokers married to husbands who smoke, in comparison with those whose husbands did not smoke. Although the RR of Japanese female active smokers was 3.8, the amount of lung cancer attributable to passive smoking in women was potentially greater than from active smoking in Japan because there were four times as many women exposed to passive smoke as there were active smoking women. In a hospital-based case control study, in Greece, Trichopoulos et al. (1981) reported almost identical findings.

These early studies were greeted with some skepticism because of the potential for misclassification of smoking status. It would only be necessary for a few active female smokers to be misclassified as nonsmokers for the effects observed to be produced. The potential for this was particularly great in Hirayama's study as it was not as socially acceptable for women to smoke in Japan in 1966, when the data were collected, as is now the case. However, any such misclassification would lead to underestimation of the relative risk.

Publication of the early results led to a succession of studies. Some were largely negative (Kabat and Wynder 1984; Koo et al. 1985). An examination of the data from the large American Cancer Society cohort study was also negative (Garfinkel 1981). Part of the difficulty related to the overwhelming importance of active smoking in the etiology of lung cancer, and the rarity of lung cancer in nonsmokers. Thus, in order to obtain sufficient subjects in a case-control study, Garfinkel et al. (1985) had to identify cases from four hospitals over an 11-year period. Patients with colorectal cancer served as controls. A significantly increased risk was found for nonsmoking women with husbands who smoked 40 or more cigarettes a day, or 20 or more at home. This excess risk was largely restricted to cases with squamous cell carcinoma.

A case-control study based on the atomic bomb survivors in Japan (Akiba et al. 1986) recently demonstrated results similar to the original reports by Hirayama (1981) and Trichopoulos et al. (1981). Specifically, the RR for nonsmoking women married to husbands who smoked 30 or more cigarettes a day relative to women married to nonsmoking husbands was 2.1, with a 95% confidence interval (CI) ranging from 0.7 to 2.5.

Excess risk for cases with histological types recognized as being strongly smoking related, such as squamous or small cell carcinomas rather than adenocarcinomas, has been found in a number of other studies, adding to the biological plausibility of the association. Thus, Dalager et al. (1986), in a joint analysis of the results of two case-control studies in the United States, found that the RR for the occurrence of squamous and small-cell carcinomas in nonsmoking women married to smoking husbands was 2.88 (95% CI 0.91–9.10), for adenocarcinoma 1.02 (0.33–3.16) and for other histological types 1.31 (0.48–3.57), women married to nonsmoking husbands being the referent. A similar effect was found in a nested case-control study set within a cohort of 27409 nonsmoking Swedish women identified from questionnaires mailed in 1961 and 1963 (Pershagen et al. 1987). In this study it was possible to examine the effect of both intensity of husbands smoking and histological type simultaneously. The RR for occurrence of squamous or small-celled carcinoma among nonsmoking women married to husbands who smoked 15 or more cigarettes a day was 6.4 (1.1–34.7). The RR for occurrence of other histological types with husbands who smoked with similar intensity was 2.4 (0.6–8.7), nonsmoking women married to nonsmoking husbands being the referent.

Wald et al. (1986) carried out a meta-analysis of 13 studies of passive smoking and lung cancer. There was a consistent tendency for excess risk to be seen from passive smoking. The conjoint risk from ten case-control studies was 1.27 (1.05–1.53) and from three cohort studies 1.44 (1.20–1.72), the latter being heavily influenced by Hirayama's results. For all 13 studies the RR was 1.35 (1.19–1.54). Adjustment for misclassification reduced this risk to 1.30, but adjustment for the fact that the referents (largely nonsmoking women married to nonsmoking husbands) were in fact exposed to some passive smoking from others raised the RR to 1.53.

Drawing on the data base on passive smoking, Wigle et al. (1987a,b) recently estimated the number of lung cancer deaths in Canada due to involuntary smoking. Using methods similar to those described previously for active smoking, it was estimated that a total of about 50–60 lung cancer deaths each year may be due to spousal smoking. For environmental tobacco smoke in general, it was estimated that a total of about 330 deaths may be due to passive smoking.

Saccharin

Saccharin, an artificial sweetener widely used prior to the introduction of aspartame, is carcinogenic to the male rat bladder, but has failed to produce consistent and convincing evidence of being able to induce cancer in humans (Arnold et al. 1983). High levels of dietary saccharin induce bladder cancer in rats give the artificial sweetener from conception to parturition to death using the two-generation testing protocol involving exposure in utero or from immediately after parturition to death (Arnold and Clayson 1985; Schoenig et al. 1985). However, the relatively large scale study conducted by the International Research Development Corporation failed to resolve the uncertainties as to the level of risk associated with low levels of exposure (Schoenig et al. 1985).

Artificial sweeteners have been the subject of extensive epidemiological investigation (Armstrong 1985), including temporal trend studies, studies of diabetics, and case-control studies. Although studies of overall trends in bladder cancer mortality have been interpreted as being negative, such studies are of limited value due to the small proportion of the general population exposed to large quantities of artificial sweeteners (saccharin and cyclamate), and to the uncertain influences of other known risk factors for bladder carcinogenesis such as smoking and occupation. Changes in diagnostic criteria and methods of treatment may also affect the interpretation of such longitudinal data.

Because of their greater consumption of artificial sweeteners, diabetic populations have been selected for study in several investigations. Although clearly negative, such studies did not monitor artificial sweetener consumption on an individual basis, and could not control for the possible effects of smoking and other risk factors for bladder cancer.

Armstrong (1985) reviewed 13 case-control studies involving artificial sweeteners conducted between 1974 and 1982. One further study has since been reported (Mommsen et al. 1983). In general, these studies were largely unable to distinguish between the use of saccharin and cyclamate, and could be subject to some degree of recall bias. Selection bias may also occur in studies using hospital controls if the disease status of these control patients was related to the use of artificial sweeteners (Silverman et al. 1983).

Taken as a whole, these results provide little evidence that saccharin induces neoplastic change in the urinary bladder in humans (Cordle and Miller 1984). Nonetheless, Howe et al. (1977) reported a significant increase in the relative risk of bladder cancer in males using artificial sweetener. In contrast, Hoover and Strasser (1980) noted elevated risks only in selected population subgroups, such as nonsmoking white females otherwise at low risk from bladder cancer.

The toxicological and epidemiological data on saccharin have been the subject of a series of reviews conducted by a number of national and international organizations (Arnold and Krewski 1988), without reaching a firm position as to the status of this compound. Reconciliation of the toxicological and epidemiological evidence on the carcinogenic potential of saccharin was attempted at a symposium sponsored by the International Agency for Research on Cancer (Wald and Doll 1985). The consensus of opinion among the participants at this meeting was that the epidemiological data were, on balance, of greater relevance to the human situation. However, although it was concluded that "saccharin, used either alone or in combination with cyclamates, is not a demonstrable cause of bladder cancer in the human population at large under past conditions of use", it was noted that the possibility of a weak effect could not be completely excluded (Krewski 1985) as in the previous review conducted by the IARC (1982).

The dilemmas posed by this artificial sweetener may possibly arise from the fact that the level of human exposure is too low to elicit an epidemiologically detectable effect. However, at present the possibility can not be excluded that the mechanism of action of saccharin is such that certain subgroups of the human population may be at risk. This seems to be the case in rats where exposure beginning immediately postpartum, or after certain toxic insults to the urothelium, appears to be critical. Resolution of this problem would be greatly facilitated if the carcinogenic mechanism of saccharin in rats could be resolved (Clayson 1984).

Formaldehyde

Formaldehyde is a colourless gas with a pungent suffocating odor. It is ubiquitous in the environment, due to release from both natural and man-made sources, and is present in the body at low levels. Formaldehyde has long been recognized to be a sensory irritant in humans (Meek et al. 1988). More recently, it has been found to be carcinogenic in animals. Several epidemiological studies have been conducted to investigate the possibility that formaldehyde may be also carcinogenic in humans.

Formaldehyde has been carcinogenic in two strains of rats, producing a high incidence of nasal tumours following inhalation exposure of 15 ppm 6 h/day 5 days/week over a 2-year period (Swenberg et al. 1980; Albert et al. 1982). In mice, nasal tumours have also been observed at 15 ppm (Kerns et al. 1983), although the increase was not statistically significant and was restricted to one sex. Studies with hamsters have provided no indication of carcinogenic effects (Dalbey 1982). There is currently no evidence that formaldehyde increases the incidence of tumours at sites other than the nasal cavity.

These toxicological findings of carcinogenicity in laboratory animals were followed by an extensive series of epidemiological investigations, including several historical cohort studies (IARC 1987). In none of these studies was there any clearly significant excess of nasal or nasopharnygeal cancer associated with exposure to formaldehyde (Meek et al. 1988). For example, Acheson et al. (1984a) reported increased mortality due to lung, rectal, bone and thyroid tumours in British chemical workers in comparison with the British population as a whole. However, these increases were not apparent when local residents were used as the basis for comparison. There was also little evidence of a dose-response relationship, rendering an association with formaldehyde exposure improbable (Acheson et al. 1984b).

Blair et al. (1986) studied 26000 workers in industrial facilities producing or using formaldehyde. Although an excess of Hodgkin's disease and cancer of the lung and prostate was noted, these effects were not consistently related to exposure level and duration. An increasing gradient in standardized mortality ratios was noted with exposure to formaldehyde in five workers with nasopharyngeal cancer who were also exposed to particulate matter (Blair et al. 1987). This latter analysis has been criticized by Collins et al. (1987), who raised questions concerning the consistency of these results, the measurement of particulate exposure, the short duration of employment of some of the cases, and the use of indirect rather than direct standardization to compare exposure groups.

The association between exposure to formaldehyde and nasal or nasopharyngeal cancer has been addressed in a series of ten case-control studies (IARC 1987; Meek et al. 1988). In a study of Scandanavian workers conducted by Hernberg et al. (1983), a possible association between formaldehyde exposure and nasal cancer was strongly confounded by exposure to wood dust. Vaughan et al. (1986) noted a significant association between cancer of the nasopharynx and residence in a mobile home for 10 years or more. However, these investigators were cautious in their interpretation of this finding, since it is based on a small number of cases and may be due to factors other than formaldehyde.

Hayes et al. (1986) examined 116 male cases of nasal and paranasal sinus tumours and corresponding controls with respect to occupational exposure to formaldehyde. After adjusting for smoking habits and exposure to wood dust, the *RR* for squamous cell carcinomas due to exposure to formaldehyde appeared to be elevated. However, the authors did not consider these results as providing conclusive evidence of formaldehyde carcinogenicity due to limitations in assessing formaldehyde exposure.

An association between formaldehyde exposure and tumour occurrence at sites other than the nasal cavity has been observed in several of the proportionate mortality studies conducted to date (Walrath and Fraumeni 1983; Liebling et al. 1984; Stayner et al. 1985). However, these results add little to the weight of evidence concerning the carcinogenicity of formaldehyde because of the potential for bias in these studies. These findings have also not been corroborated in the cohort and case-control studies discussed above.

Taken as a whole, the evidence of the carcinogenicity of formaldehyde in human populations in epidemiological studies conducted to date is not conclusive (UAREP 1988). Slight increases in cancer at several sites, including the lung and nasal cavity, have been reported in some cohort and case-control studies. However, these results should be interpreted with caution due to inconsistencies between studies and the absence of an increase in risk with increasing duration of and level of exposure to formaldehyde. Limitations in exposure ascertainment and potential confounding with other risk factors such as particulate matter and wood dust also complicate the interpretation of the results. Nonetheless, the International Agency for Research on Cancer (IARC 1987) and the U.S. Environmental Protection Agency (EPA 1987) have recently concluded that the epidemiological data provide "limited" evidence of the carcinogenicity of formaldehyde in humans, according to their criteria for classifying the weight of evidence for carcinogenicity based on epidemiological data.

Weight of Evidence for Carcinogenicity

The existence of a series of well-conducted epidemiological and toxicological studies yielding consistently strong evidence of carcinogenicity leaves little doubt concerning the test agent's ability to induce neoplastic changes. In other instances, however, the available data will be less clear cut. This can occur when the effects seen are equivocal, or when inconsistencies between studies of a similar nature occur. Discrepancies between laboratory findings and human observations can also raise questions as to whether the toxicological results predict risks to humans which are difficult to detect epidemiologically, or whether the animal data are not relevant due to species differences in response or exposure conditions. While prudence would suggest that the epidemiological studies may simply be insensitive, the possibility that humans are genuinely resistant to the effects observed in animals cannot be wholly discounted, particularly in the presence of an extensive series of sound human studies revealing no effects (Wald and Doll 1985). Such a conclusion should be supported by sound mechanistic evidence explaining why such discrepancies exist.

In this regard, it has, until recently, generally been assumed that a carcinogen demonstrable in experimental animals will ipso facto be effective in humans and that, because carcinogenesis is a stochastic process, it is not possible to devise a safe exposure level of such an agent for humans. An examination of all the toxicological evidence may sometimes suggest that these assumptions are not necessarily valid. For example, the use of animals with a moderate to high background incidence of tumours in a specific tissue, or the use of levels of the test agent that induce toxicity in one or more tissues, may confound the direct application of a particular bioassay to humans (Clayson 1987). In such cases it is necessary to carefully evaluate the epidemiological and toxicological data to ensure that the overall evidence supports the conclusion that the animal data are not relevant to humans. Further work to explain why a particular toxicological result is most unlikely to be of human relevance will be of basic importance, as illustrated in the recent case of butylated hydroxyanisole (BHA) (Clayson et al. 1986; Iverson et al. 1985). In this case, the cellular proliferation which precedes tumorigenesis in the rat is not detectable at the low levels of exposure to which humans are subjected.

A related issue is the level of evidence required to conclude reasonably that an agent is not carcinogenic to animals or humans. Even with well-conducted studies that are apparently negative, there can be no absolute assurance that the agent of interest possesses no carcinogenic potential (Clayson and Krewski 1986). This reflects the statistical limitations in sensitivity inherent in studies involving only a sample of subjects rather than the entire population at risk (Day 1985; Krewski et al. 1988b). Since the denial of negative results in this fashion would preclude the rational regulation of carcinogens, the existence of a convincing body of negative toxicological and epidemiological data is taken to provide adequate assurance that the substance of interest will not present an appreciable risk.

A logical conclusion of such considerations is the need for criteria to evaluate the weight of evidence for carcinogenicity. In this regard, the International Agency for Research on Cancer has established categories of evidence for carcinogenicity based on bioassay results (IARC 1987). Sufficient evidence of carcinogenicity in animals is comprised of positive results either in two or more species or in two or more independent studies; an exceptionally high rate of occurrence of neoplasms in a single strain or study may also suffice. Limited evidence of carcinogenicity occurs when positive results are observed only in a single experiment, when only benign neoplasms are involved, or when unresolved questions about the data remain. Inadequate evidence exists when the bioassay results cannot be interpreted because of study limitations. The final category of carcinogenicity requires no evidence of carcinogenic effects in at least two species.

IARC (1987) also classifies human carcinogenicity data using categories similar to those used to classify animal evidence. When studies indicate a positive relationship in which chance, bias and confounding effects can be ruled out, there is sufficient evidence of carcinogenicity. If a positive relationship is found but such effects cannot be ruled out, evidence is limited. Several adequate studies which provide mutually consistent evidence not showing a positive association at relevant exposure levels provide evidence suggesting lack of carcinogenicity. If the available studies are judged to be of insufficient quality, consistency or statistical power, there is inadequate evidence of carcinogenicity.

These two schemes may be combined to arrive at an overall evaluation of the weight of evidence for carcinogenicity (IARC 1987). When there is sufficient human evidence of carcinogenesis, an agent is considered carcinogenic to humans (group 1). An agent with limited human evidence and sufficient animal evidence is considered probably carcinogenic to humans (group 2A); in the absence of sufficient animal evidence, the same agent is considered possibly carcinogenic to humans (group 2B). In contrast to the preceding proposal, a combination of animal and human evidence suggesting a lack of carcinogenicity is required for an agent to be designated as probably not carcinogenic to humans (group 4). Agents which do not fall into Groups 1, 2 or 4 are not classified with respect to their carcinogenicity to humans (group 3).

Applying these criteria, saccharin falls into group 2B on the basis of inconclusive human evidence but sufficient animal evidence of carcinogenicity (IARC 1987). Formaldehyde falls into group 2A, with limited human evidence and sufficient animal evidence of carcinogenicity. Only one chemical – caprolactam – presently falls into group 4. Tobacco smoke falls into group 1 since there is sufficient evidence of its carcinogenicity in humans in active smokers. Although the epidemiologic evidence on passive smoking is consistent with either an increased cancer risk or an absence of risk, the IARC (1986, 1987) has concluded that involuntary smoking may give rise to some risk of cancer. Nonetheless, further epidemiologic research on passive smoking would be useful in clarifying this situation.

Ultimately, the effective melding of epidemiological and toxicological data to provide a framework for public health protection demands an adequate knowledge of the mechanisms that lead to cancer. Schemata such as these proposed by NTP (1985), EPA (1986) and IARC (1987) do little more than assume that certain epidemiologically or toxicologically determined facts have a specific significance. The recent emergence of the sciences of molecular biology, pharmacokinetics, genotoxicology and immunotoxicology hold the promise of replacing assumption by factual knowledge in assessing the meaning of toxicological studies with reference to public health.

Summary and Conclusions

Human health risk assessment has been the object of systematic study in recent years, with formal models of risk assessment and risk management having been proposed by several national and international health agencies. The particular model developed by the Environmental Health Directorate of Health and

Welfare Canada was examined in some detail and used to focus on the role of epidemiology in the overall process of risk assessment. In addition to providing information fundamental to the identification of environmental carcinogens and the estimation of carcinogenic risks, epidemiology may also play a role in shaping risk preception and in improving risk communication practices.

Taken collectively, epidemiologic data on health risks provide a basis for improved disease surveillance and prioritization of public health concerns. Both descriptive and analytic epidemiologic protocols may be used to gather information on disease etiology. Because of the potential for bias and confounding in observational studies of human populations, epidemiological data should be subjected to careful evaluation in accordance with established criteria before a causal relationship between exposure and disease is inferred. Toxicological studies using nonhuman test systems may be used to avoid these problems, but at the expense of obtaining indirect information on human health risks. Nonetheless, toxicological data provide an important complement to epidemiological data, providing information on potential health risks in advance of human exposure and offering a means of indirectly assessing risks in situations where human studies fail to provide informative results.

The complementary roles of epidemiology and toxicology in health risk assessment were examined using four case studies. While the epidemiological evidence linking tobacco consumption to lung cancer is now unequivocal, the corresponding data on involuntary smoking, although strongly suggestive of increasing the relative risk of lung cancer, requires further confirmation before providing the same degree of evidence as now exists for active smoking. At present, the best estimates suggest that overall mortality attributable to active smoking may exceed that due to passive smoking by roughly 100-fold. Despite this large difference in health impact, passive smoking continues to be the focus of much public concern, in part because of the involuntary nature of the risk involved.

Because of the abundance of good epidemiological data on tobacco, toxicology has assumed a secondary role in defining the health risks associated with smoking. In contrast, while epidemiological studies with saccharin and formaldehyde have provided less clear-cut evidence of adverse health effects in humans, laboratory studies have provided unequivocal evidence of carcinogenic effects in animals exposed to high doses, thereby raising concerns over potential human carcinogenicity.

In assessing conflicting epidemiological and toxicological evidence, consideration needs to be given to the fact that human studies may, for various reasons, be unable to detect effects seen in nonhuman test systems. In this regard, classification schemes based on the combined weight of evidence for carcinogenicity derived from animal and human studies may be used to arrive at a position on the potential for the agent of interest to induce cancer in humans. At the same time, the possibility that effects seen in animals at high doses may not be relevant to humans exposed to lower doses cannot be completely dismissed. Resolution of such differences will however require a clear understanding of the mechanism by which such agents exert their carcinogenic effects in animals and humans.

References

Acheson ED, Barnes HR, Gardner MJ, Osmond C, Pannett B, Taylor CP (1984a) Formaldehyde in the British chemical industry. An occupational cohort study. Lancet i: 611–616

Acheson ED, Barnes HR, Gardner MJ, Osmond C, Pannett B, Taylor CP (1984b) Formaldehyde process workers and lung cancer. Lancet i: 1066–1067

Akiba S, Kato H, Blot WJ (1986) Passive smoking and lung cancer among Japanese women. Cancer Res 46: 4804–4807

Albert RE, Sellakumar AR, Laskin S, Kuschner M, Nelson N, Snyder CA (1982) Gaseous formaldehyde and hydrogen chloride induction of nasal cancer in the rat. JNCI 68: 597–603

Armstrong BK (1985) Saccharin/cyclamates: epidemiological evidence. In: Wald NJ, Doll R (eds) Interpretation of negative epidemiological evidence for carcinogenicity. International Agency for Research on Cancer, Lyon, pp 129–143 (IARC sci publ no 65)

Arnold DL, Clayson DB (1985) Saccharin – a bitter-sweet case. In: Clayson DB, Krewski D, Munro I (eds) Toxicological risk assessment, vol 2. General criteria and case studies. CRC, Boca Raton Fl, pp 227–243

Arnold DL, Krewski D (1988) Saccharin: still a controversial sweetener. In: Grima L, Fowles CD (eds) Information needs for risk management. Institute for Environmental Studies, University of Toronto (Environmental monogr no 8) pp 193–204

Arnold DL, Krewski D, Munro IC (1983) Saccharin: a toxicological and historical perspective. Toxicology 27: 179–256

Blair A, Stewart P, O'Berg M, Gaffey W, Walrath J, Ward J, Bales R, Kaplan S, Cubit D (1986) Mortality among industrial workers exposed to formaldehyde. JNCI 76: 1071–1084

Blair A, Stewart PA, Hoover RN, Fraumeni JF, Walrath J, O'Berg M, Gaffey W (1987) Cancers of the nasopharynx and oropharynx and formaldehyde exposure (letter to the editor). JNCI 78: 191–192

Breslow NE, Day NE (1980) Statistical methods in cancer research, vol 1 – the analysis of case-control studies. International Agency for Research on Cancer, Lyon (IARC sci publ no 82)

Breslow NE, Day NE (1987) Statistical methods in cancer research, vol 2 – the design and analysis of cohort studies. International Agency for Research on Cancer, Lyon (IARC sci publ no 82)

Burnett RT, Krewski D, Birkwood PL, Franklin CA (1988) Health risks from transported air pollution: a Canadian perspective. In: Fowles CD, Grima L, Munn RE (eds) Information needs for risk management. Institute for Environmental Studies, University of Toronto (Environmental monogr no 8), pp 283–290

Clayson DB (1984) The mode of carcinogenic action of saccharin. Cancer Lett 22: 119–123

Clayson DB (1987) The need for biological risk assessment in reaching decisions about carcinogens. Mutat Res 185: 243–269

Clayson DB, Krewski D (1986) The concept of negativity in experimental carcinogenesis. Mutat Res 167: 233–240
Clayson DB, Iverson F, Nera E, Lok E, Rogers C, Rodrigues C, Page D, Karpinski K (1986) Histopathological and radioautographical studies on the forestomach of F344 rats treated with butylated hydroxyanisole and related chemicals. Food Chem Toxicol 24: 1171–1182
Collins JJ, Caporossi JC, Utidijian HMD (1987) Cancers of the nasopharynx and oropharynx and formaldehyde exposure (letter to the editor). JNCI 78: 192–193
Collishaw NE, Tostowaryk W, Wigle DT (1988) Mortality attributable to tobacco to tobacco use in Canada. Can J Public Health 79: 166–169
Cordle F, Miller SA (1984) Using epidemiology to regulate food additives: saccharin case-control studies. Public Health Rep 99: 365–369
Covello V, von Winterfeldt D, Slovic P (1987) Risk communication: a review of the literature. Risk Abs 4: 171–182
Dalager NA, Pickle LW, Mason TJ, Correa P, Fontham E, Stemhagen A, Buffler PA, Ziegler RG, Fraumeni JF Jr (1986) The relation of passive smoking to lung cancer. Cancer Res 46: 4808–4811
Dalbey WE (1982) Formaldehyde and tumors in hamster respiratory tract. Toxicology 24: 9–14
Davies JC, Covello VT, Allen FW (eds) (1987) Risk communication. Conservation Foundation, Washington DC
Day NE (1985) Statistical considerations. In: Wald NJ, Doll R (eds) Interpretation of negative epidemiological evidence for carcinogenicity. International Agency for Research on Cancer, Lyon, pp 13–27 (IARC sci publ no 65)
DHHS: Department of Health and Human Services (1980) The health consequences of smoking for women: a report of the surgeon general. US Government Printing Office, Washington DC
DHSS: Department of Health and Human Services (1982) The health consequences of smoking: cancer. A report of the surgeon general. US Government Printing Office, Washington DC
Doll R, Peto R (1976) Mortality in relation to smoking: 20 years' observations on male doctors. Br Med J 2: 1525–1536
Doll R, Peto R (1981) The causes of cancer: quantitative estimates of avoidable risks of cancer in the United States today. JNCI 66: 1191–1308
EPA: Environmental Protection Agency (1986) Guidelines for carcinogen risk assessment. Fed Regist 51: 33992–34003
EPA: Environmental Protection Agency (1987) Assessment of health risks to garment workers and certain home residents from exposure to formaldehyde. Office of pesticides and toxic substances, Washington DC
Garfinkel L (1981) Time trends in lung cancer mortality among nonsmokers and a note on passive smoking. JNCI 66: 1061–1066
Garfinkel L, Auerbach O, Joubert L (1985) Involuntary smoking and lung cancer: a case-control study. JNCI 75: 463–469
Glass RI (1986) New prospects for epidemiologic investigations. Science 234: 951–955
Godley FH (1974) Cigarette smoking, social factors, and mortality: new estimates from representative national samples. PhD dissertation, University of Maryland.
Gori GB (1976) Low-risk cigarettes: a prescription. Science 194: 1243–1246
Hayes RB, Raatgever JW, DeBruyn A, Gerin M (1986) Cancer of the nasal cavity and paranasal sinuses, and formaldehyde exposure. Int J Cancer 37: 487–492

Herbst AL, Poskanzer DC, Robboy SJ, Scully RE (1975) Prenatal exposure to stilbestrol: a prospective comparison of exposed female offspring with unexposed controls. N Engl J Med 292: 334–339

Hernberg S, Westerholm P, Schulz-Larsen K, Degerth R, Kuosma E, Englund A, Engzell U, Hansen HS, Mutanen P (1983) Nasal and sinonasal cancer. Connection with occupational exposures in Denmark, Finland and Sweden. Scand J Work Environ Health 9: 315–326

Hill AB (1965) The environment and disease: association or causation? Proc R Soc Med 58: 295–380

Hill GB, Mao Y, Laidlaw J, Sanscartier GP, Silins J (eds) (1988) Canadian cancer statistics. Canadian Cancer Society, Toronto

Hirayama T (1981) Non-smoking wives of heavy smokers have a higher risk of lung cancer: a study from Japan. Br Med J (Clin Res) 282: 183–185

Hoel DG, Landrigan PJ (1987) Comprehensive evaluation of humans' data. In: Tardiff RG, Rodricks JV (eds) Toxic substances and human risk: principles of data interpretation. Plenum, New York, pp 121–130

Hoffman D, Masuda Y, Wynder EL (1969) α-Naphthylamine and β-naphthylamine in cigarette smoke. Nature 221: 255–256

Hoffman D, Adams JD, Piade JJ, Hecht SS (1980) Chemical studies on tobacco smoke LXVIII. Analysis of volatile and tobacco-specific nitrosamines in tobacco products. In: Walker EA, Castegnaro M, Griciute L, Borzsonyi M (eds) N-nitroso compounds: analysis, formation and occurrence. IARC, Lyon (IARC Scientific Publications No. 31)

Hoover RN, Strasser PH (1980) Artificial sweeteners and human bladder cancer. Preliminary results. Lancet i: 837–840

Howe GR, Burch JD, Miller AB, Morrison B, Gordon P, Weldon L, Chambers LW, Fodor G, Windsor GM (1977) Artificial sweeteners and human bladder cancer. Lancet ii: 578–581

Howe GR, Lindsay J, Coppock E, Miller AB (1979) Isoniazid exposure in relation to cancer incidence and mortality in a cohort of tuberculosis patients. Int J Epidemiol 8: 305–312

IARC: International Agency for Research on Cancer (1982) Chemicals, industrial processes and industries associated with cancer in humans. IRAC monographs, Volumes 1 to 29. IARC, Lyon (IARC monogr, suppl 4)

IARC: International Agency for Research on Cancer (1986) IARC monographs on the evaluation of the carcinogenic risk of chemicals to humans. Tobacco smoking, vol 38. IARC, Lyon

IARC: International Agency for Research on Cancer (1987) IARC monographs on the evaluation of carcinogenic risk to humans. Overall evaluations of carcinogenicity: an updating of IARC monographs volumes 1–42. IARC, Lyon.

Iverson F, Truelove J, Nera E, Wong J, Lok E, Clayson DB (1985) An 85-day study of butylated hydroxyanisole in the cynomolgus monkey. Cancer Lett 26: 43–50

Johansen H, Semenciw R, Morrison H, Mao Y, Verdier P, Smith ME, Wigle DT (1987) Important risk factors for death in adults: a 10-year follow-up of the Nutrition Canada survey cohort. Can Med Assoc J 136: 823–828

Kabat GC, Wynder EL (1984) Lung cancer in nonsmokers. Cancer 53: 1214–1221

Kerns WD, Donofrio DJ, Pavkov KL (1983) The chronic effects of formaldehyde inhalation in rats and mice: a preliminary report. In: Gibson JE (ed) Formaldehyde toxicity. Hemisphere, Washington DC, pp 111–131

Koo LC, Ho JHC, Lee N (1985) An analysis of some risk factors for lung cancer in Hong Kong. Int J Cancer 35: 149–155
Krewski D (1985) Saccharin/cyclamates: conclusion. In: Wald NJ, Doll R (eds) Interpretation of negative epidemiological evidence for carcinogenicity. IARC, Lyon, pp 145–148
Krewski D (1987) Risk and risk management: issues and approaches. In: McColl RS (ed) Environmental health risks: assessment and management. University of Waterloo Press, Waterloo, pp 29–51
Krewski D, Birkwood PL (1987) Risk assessment and risk management. Risk Abs 4: 53–61
Krewski D, Birkwood PL (1988) Regulatory and nonregulatory options for risk management. In: Martin LRG, Lafond G (eds) Risk management: estimation, evaluation and assessment. University of Waterloo Press, Waterloo, pp 253–271
Krewski D, Somers E, Birkwood PL (1987) Risk perception in a decision-making context. Carcinog Rev 5: 175–209
Krewski D, Goddard MJ, Murdoch D (1989a) Statistical consideration in the interpretation of negative carcinogenicity data. Regul Toxicol Pharmacol 9: 5–22
Krewski D, Oxman A, Torrance GW (1989b) A decision oriented framework for evaluating environmental risk management strategies: a case study of lead in gasoline. In: Paustenbach DJ (eds) Environmental risk assessment: a textbook of case studies. Wiley, New York, pp 1047–1062
Leiss W, Krewski D (1989) Risk communication: theory and practice. In: Leiss W (ed) Prospects and problems in risk communication. University of Waterloo Press, Waterloo, pp 89–112
Liebling T, Rosenman KD, Pastides H, Griffith RG, Lemeshow S (1984) Cancer mortality among workers exposed to formaldehyde. Am J Ind Med 5: 423–428
Magnus K (1982) Trends in cancer incidence: causes and practical implications. Hemisphere, Washington DC
Mao Y, Smith MH (1983) The lung cancer epidemic among Canadian women. Chronic Dis Can 4: 33–35
Mao Y, Smith H, Simpson H (1982) Recent mortality trends of leading causes of death in Canada. Chronic Dis Can 3: 19–21
Meek ME, Krewski D, Birkwood PL (1988) Formaldehyde: science, regulation and information needs. In: Grima L, Fowles CD (eds) Information needs for risk management. Institute for Environmental Studies, University of Toronto (in press) (Environmental monogr no 8)
Miller AB (1984) The information explosion – the role of the epidemiologist. Cancer Forum 8: 67–75
Mommsen S, Aagaard J, Sell A (1983) A case-control study of female bladder cancer. Eur J Cancer Clin Oncol 19: 725–729
Newcombe HB (1967) Record linkage: the design of efficient systems for linking records into individual and family histories. Am J Hum Genet 19: 335–359
Pershagen G, Hrubec Z, Svensson C (1987) Passive smoking and lung cancer in Swedish women. Am J Epidemiol 125: 17–24
Rothman KJ, Keller AZ (1972) The effect of joint exposure to alcohol and tobacco on risk of cancer of the mouth and pharynx. J Chronic Dis 25: 711–716
Saracci R (1987) The interactions of tobacco smoking and other agents in cancer etiology. Epidemiol Rev 9: 175–193
Schoenig GP, Goldenthal EI, Geil RG, Frith CH, Richter WR, Carlborg FW (1985)

Evaluation of the dose response and in utero exposure to saccharin in the rat. Food Chem Toxicol 23: 475–490
Schottenfeld D, Fraumeni JF (1982) Cancer epidemiology and prevention. Saunders, Philadelphia
Selikoff IJ, Hammond EC (1975) Multiple risk factors in environmental cancer. In: Fraumeni JF Jr (ed) Persons at high risk of cancer: an approach to cancer etiology and control. Academic, New York, pp 467–483
Sies H (1988) A new parameter for sex education. Nature 332: 495
Silverman DT, Hoover RN, Swanson GM (1983) Artificial sweetners and lower urinary tract cancer: hospital vs population controls. Am J Epidemiol 117: 326–334
Somers E (1983) Environmental health risk management in Canada. Regul Toxicol Pharmacol 3: 75–81
Somers E (1984) Risk estimation for environmental chemicals as a basis for decision making. Regul Toxicol Pharmacol 4: 99–106
Stayner L, Smith AB, Reeve G, Blade L, Elliott L, Keenlyside R, Halperin W (1985) Proportionate mortality study of workers in the garment industry exposed to formaldehyde. Am J Ind Med 7: 229–240
Swenberg JA, Kerns WD, Mitchell RI, Gralla EJ, Pavkov KL (1980) Induction of squamous cell carcinomas of the rat nasal cavity by inhalation exposure to formaldehyde vapor. Cancer Res 40: 3398–3402
Torrance GW, Krewski D (1985) Economic evaluation of toxic chemical control programs. Toxic Substances J 7: 53–71
Trichopoulos D, Kalandidi A, Sparros L, MacMahon B (1981) Lung cancer and passive smoking. Int J Cancer 27: 1–4
UAREP: Universities Associated for Research and Education in Pathology (1988) Epidemiology of chronic occupational exposure to formaldehyde: report of the ad hoc panel on health aspects of formaldehyde. Toxicol Ind Health 4: 77–90
Vaughan TL, Strader C, Davis S, Daling JR (1986) Formaldehyde and cancers of the pharynx, sinus, and nasal cavity: II. Residential exposures. Int J Cancer 38: 685–688
Veterans Administration Coronary Artery Bypass Surgery Cooperative Study Group (1984) Eleven-year survival in the veterans administration randomized trial of coronary bypass surgery for stable angina. N Engl J Med 311: 1333–1339
Wald N, Doll R (eds) (1985) Interpretation of negative epidemiological evidence for carcinogenicity. IARC, Lyon
Wald NJ, Nanchahal K, Thompson SG, Cuckle HS (1986) Does breathing other people's tobacco smoke cause lung cancer? Br Med J 293: 1217–1222
Walrath J, Fraumeni JF (1983) Mortality patterns among embalmers. Int J Cancer 31: 407–411
WHO: World Health Organization (1985) Risk management in chemical safety. WHO European Regional Program on Chemical Safety, Geneva
Wigle DT, Mao Y, Grace M (1980) Relative importance of smoking as a risk factor for selected cancers. Can J Public Health 71: 269–275
Wigle DT (1984) Public health enemy no 1: smoking. Can Pharm J 117: 140–144, 146
Wigle DT (1985) Early evidence that smoking causes lung cancer. Chronis Dis Can 6: 41–42
Wigle DT, Mao Y, Semenciw R, Morrison HI (1986) Cancer patterns in Canada. Can Med Assoc J 134: 231–235
Wigle DT, Collishaw NE, Kirkbride J, Mao Y (1987a) Deaths in Canada from lung cancer due to involuntary smoking. Can Med Assoc J 136: 945–951

Wigle DT, Collishaw NE, Kirkbride J (1987b) Exposure of involuntary smokers to toxic components of tobacco smoke. Can J Public Health 78: 151–154
Working Group on Risk Assessment and Risk Management (1988) Risk assessment/risk management: a handbook for use with the Bureau of Chemical Hazards. Environmental Health Directorate, Health and Welfare Canada, Ottawa
Wynder GL, Hoffmann D (1982) Tobacco. In: Schottenfeld D, Fraumeni JF Jr (eds) Cancer epidemiology and prevention. Saunders, Philadelphia, pp 277–292

Discovering Occupational Carcinogens in Population-Based Case-Control Studies: Review of Findings from an Exposure-Based Approach and a Methodologic Comparison of Alternative Data Collection Strategies

J. Siemiatycki

Epidemiology and Preventive Medicine Research Center, Institut Armand-Frappier, 531 Boulevard des Prairies, Laval, Quebec H7N 4Z3, Canada

Introduction

The identification of environmental carcinogens is one of the main public health problems of our era. Many, if not most known carcinogens are occupational exposures (Doll and Peto 1981). There are two reasons for this. It is much easier to identify persons as having a common occupation or occupational exposure than it is to identify them as having common exposure to a dietary, atmospheric, psychosocial, or other type of environment. Also, the work environment has tended to be more polluted than the domestic or general environment. However, of the thousands of substances to which workers are exposed in the workplace, only a handful have ever been assessed in epidemiologic studies for carcinogenic potential. It is reasonable to suspect that many occupational carcinogens have not yet been discovered. Considering the enormous number of chemical and physical agents in the workplace, what kind of epidemiologic monitoring approach can be applied to the problem to flag potential carcinogens?

Discovering occupational hazards requires the juxtaposition of two sets of data: information on illness or death among workers and information on their occupations, industries, and/or occupational conditions. A third, optional data set which would improve the validity of inferences drawn from that juxtaposition is the set of nonoccupational risk factors which may confound the relation between occupation and disease. The more detailed and valid the information, the greater the chance of finding true associations. Insofar as occupational carcinogens are concerned, it is information on chemical and physical exposures which is desirable, especially concerning exposure incurred many years before the onset of cancer. Most studies of occupational cancer, irrespective of the study design, have been based on analysis of job or industry titles. While such analyses can be useful, job titles, whether based on a national classification or on a company scale, may be inadequate as indicators of occupational exposures. Even within a company, a given job title typically covers a group of workers whose activities and chemical exposures are heterogeneous. The variation in exposures when workers are grouped by common job

Recent Results in Cancer Research, Vol. 120

titles across industries and eras can be very substantial. Thus, a risk may go undetected because only a subset of a category may have been exposed to a carcinogen and the dilution may blur the association. For a product which is used by subsets of several occupational categories, considerable statistical power is lost if those workers with common exposure cannot be pooled. If workers could be categorized on the basis of common exposure rather than common job title, the contrasts would be sharper and relevant sample sizes larger.

For several years my research team has been carrying out a large population-based case-control study in Montreal, focusing on occupational exposures as potential risk factors (Siemiatycki et al. 1981; Siemiatycki 1984). Several sites of cancer were included in the study, the main ones being: esophagus, stomach, colorectum, liver, pancreas, lung, prostate, bladder, kidney, melanoma of the skin, and lymphoid tissue. Eligible subjects were those incident cases of any of these cancer sites, among males aged 35–70 years and resident in the Montreal area. Cases were ascertained from the 19 largest hospitals in the Montreal area. Between 1979 and 1985 interviews were carried out for 3726 cancer patients (response rate 82%). There were also interviews with 533 population controls (response rate 70%).

The in-depth interview elicited a detailed job history of each subject and information on potentially confounding covariables. A specially trained team of chemists and hygienists examined each completed questionnaire and translated each job into a list of potential exposures. They did this on a checklist which explicitly listed some 300 of the most common occupational exposures in Montreal. For each product thought to be present in each job, the chemists noted their confidence that the exposure actually occurred (possible, probable, definite), frequency of exposure during a normal workweek ($< 5\%$, 5%–30%, and $> 30\%$), and the level of concentration of the agent in the work environment (low, medium, high). Details of the exposure coding method have been described by Gérin et al. (1985) and Gérin (this volume). This data bank has already been exploited to describe associations between many occupational exposures and several types of cancer and to assess a number of methodologic issues.

The purpose of this communication is twofold: to briefly list some of our more important substantive results to date and to review some of our methodologic findings with particular emphasis on those which elucidate the value of our approach as compared with some other plausible research designs.

Review of Substantive Results to Date

Each cancer group listed above constitutes a case series which can be investigated in relation to each of the exposures in our data bank. Furthermore, there are sufficient numbers of lung cancers that the histologic subtypes could each be analysed as separate case series. For each case series, controls could be selected among other cancer sites or among population controls. Until now, we have used only the "cancer control" strategy, though in the future we will compare results using cancer controls and population controls. Thus, each subject could serve as a case in one analysis and as a control in others. The criteria for selecting controls among the other cancers and a discussion of the implications of using cancer controls have been presented elsewhere (Siemiatycki et al. 1987b).

Table 1 lists the main cancer site groups which were included in the study along with the numbers of cases and corresponding numbers of controls. Heretofore our strategy has been to focus on a small group of substances on the checklist and analyse each such group in turn. Table 2 shows the five groups of substances that have been the objects of distinct analyses and reports.

The results which are summarized here were based on intensive and exhaustive analyses that took into account hundreds of potential confounders, both occupational and nonoccupational. Multistage analyses beginning with the Mantel-Haenzsel approach for identifying promising associations and potential

Table 1. Types of cancer analyzed as case series, sites excluded from the reference series, and numbers of cases and referents

Cancer case series	Cancer sites excluded[a] from control series	Cases (*n*)	Controls (*n*)
Esophagus	Lung, stomach	107	2514
Stomach	Lung, esophagus	250	2514
Colon	Lung, other colorectal	364	2081
Rectosigmoid	Lung, other colorectal	233	2081
Rectum	Lung, other colorectal	190	1315
Liver	Lung	50	2806
Pancreas	Lung	117	2741
Lung – oat cell	Other lung	159	1523
Lung – squamous cell	Other lung	359	1523
Lung – adenocarcinoma	Other lung	162	1523
Lung – other cell types[b]	Other lung	177	1523
Prostate	Lung	452	1733
Bladder	Lung, kidney	486	2196
Kidney	Lung, bladder	181	2196
Melanoma of skin	Lung	121	2737
Hodgkin's lymphoma	Lung, other lymphoma	53	2599
Non-Hodgkin's lymphoma	Lung, Hodgkin's	206	2599

[a] For each case series, all cancer patients interviewed served as referents with the exceptions listed in this column. Furthermore, for rectum, lung, and prostate, only those subjects interviewed during the same ascertainment periods as the three respective site series were used as referents.

[b] This is a heterogeneous grouping which includes large cell, spindle cell, and adenosquamous carcinoma and "carcinoma, not otherwise specified".

Table 2. Groups of substances that have undergone intensive analysis

Group (Reference)	Substances analysed
Organic dusts[a] (Siemiatycki et al. 1986)	Wood dust; grain dust; flour dust; fabrics dust; cotton dust; wool fibers; synthetics dust; fur dust
Petroleum-derived liquids (Siemiatycki et al. 1987a)	Automotive gasoline; aviation gas; mineral spirits; kerosene; jet fuel; diesel fuel; heating oil; cutting fluids; hydraulic fluids; lubricating oils; other mineral oil; crude oil
Exhausts and combustion products (Siemiatycki et al. 1988)	Gasoline exhaust; diesel exhaust; jet fuel exhaust; propane exhaust; propane combustion; natural gas combustion; liquid fuels combustion; wood combustion; coal combustion; coke combustion
Inorganic dusts (Siemiatycki et al. 1989a)	Silica; excavation dust; concrete; cement dust; brick dust; gypsum; lime; abrasives; alumina; silicon carbide
Formaldehyde (Gérin et al. 1989)	Formaldehyde

[a] Analysis based on first 2180 subjects interviewed.

confounders and the logistic regression approach for estimating "adjusted" odds ratios were carried out (Siemiatycki et al. 1987b).

With several sites of cancer (Table 1) and 42 substances (Table 2), hundreds of associations have been evaluated, each one at different levels and durations of exposure. We have chosen to present here those associations which, in our data, provide the strongest evidence of an effect. We used information on strength of association, statistical significance, and dose-response pattern. For each association we estimated the odds ratio corresponding to any exposure (i.e., any level for any duration) and corresponding to subgroups defined by less or more than 10 years duration and by less or more than the median of a semiquantitative index of degree of exposure composed of the concentration, frequency and confidence levels. Exposure for more than 10 years at the high level of the index we call "high-long" exposure. Of all the associations, we selected for presentation those which: had at least seven exposed cases, were statistically significant at the high-long exposure level, and had at least as high an odds ratio (OR) in the high-long category as in the any exposure category. A few associations are included which did not quite meet these criteria but which we considered interesting in the light of current hypotheses or controversies.

Tables 3 through 6 present these noteworthy results based on the indepth analyses carried out to date. Table 3 shows the associations with sites of the gastrointestinal tract; Table 4 shows the associations with lung cancer and

Table 3. Noteworthy associations between gastrointestinal cancers and the substances thus far analysed

Site	Substance	Exposure Level	n^a	OR[b]	90% CI
Stomach	Wood dust	Any	55	1.8	1.3–2.6
		Long-high	18	1.9	1.2–3.0
Stomach	Gasoline	Any	44	1.6	1.1–2.3
		Long-high	11	2.3	1.2–4.2
Colorectum	Synthetic fibers	Any	34	2.1	1.2–3.6
		Long-high	16	3.0	1.6–5.7
Colon	Grain dust	Any	22	1.6	1.1–2.5
		Long-high	8	1.9	1.0–4.0
Colon	Diesel exhaust	Any	68	1.3	1.0–1.7
		Long-high	30	1.7	1.2–2.5
Rectum	Gasoline exhaust	Any	89	1.3	1.0–1.7
		Long-high	36	1.6	1.1–2.3
Rectum	Heating oil	Any	11	1.4	0.7–2.7
		Long-high	8	2.6	1.2–5.5
Pancreas	Coal combustion	Any	10	1.9	1.0–3.6
		Long-high	8	3.5	1.7–7.3

[a] Number of exposed cases.
[b] Odds ratio adjusted for many confounders.
CI, confidence interval.

histologic types of lung cancer; Table 5 shows associations with sites of the genitourinary tract; and Table 6 shows associations with lymphoma. There were no noteworthy associations with skin melanoma.

This is not the place to discuss the merits of each association presented here. Each must be evaluated on its own, taking account of the strength of evidence from our data, as well as any supporting epidemiologic or experimental data, information on route of entry, metabolism, fate of the substance, and any other relevant information. Of course there will be many false positives in any such systematic monitoring scheme. This should not be an excuse for dismissing these findings (Thomas et al. 1985). We believe that each one deserves the same consideration as any soundly based hypothesis.

Given our results and information from other epidemiological or experimental evidence, the associations which we find most plausible and important to evaluate are: stomach–wood dust; stomach–gasoline; colorectum–synthetic fibers; lung–wood dust; lung (nonadenocarcinoma)–silica dust; lung (squamous cell)–mineral spirits; lung (squamous cell)–gasoline exhaust and diesel exhaust;

Table 4. Noteworthy associations between lung cancer and the substances thus far analysed

Site	Substance	Exposure level	n[a]	OR[b]	90% CI
Lung – all	Wood dust	Any	144	1.2	1.0–1.6
		Long-high	46	1.7	1.1–2.6
Lung – non-adenocarcinoma	Silica	Any	161	1.2	1.0–1.6
		Long-high	55	1.6	1.1–2.4
Lung – non-adenocarcinoma	Excavation dust	Any	70	1.4	1.0–1.8
		Long-high	21	2.0	1.1–3.5
Lung – non-adenocarcinoma	Concrete dust	Any	58	1.2	0.8–1.6
		Long-high	27	3.4	1.9–6.1
Lung – squamous	Mineral spirits	Any	92	1.3	1.0–1.7
		Long-high	44	1.7	1.2–2.3
Lung – squamous	Diesel fuel	Any	20	1.6	1.0–2.6
		Long-high	13	2.5	1.3–4.7
Lung – squamous	Crude oil	Any	7	3.5	1.5–8.2
		Long-high	4	3.9	1.2–12.3
Lung – squamous	Gasoline exhaust	Any	182	1.2	1.0–1.5
		Long-high	76	1.4	1.1–1.8
Lung – squamous	Diesel exhaust	Any	81	1.2	0.9–1.6
		Long-high	28	1.2	0.8–1.8
Lung – oat cell	Heating oil	Any	13	1.7	1.2–3.4
		Long-high	7	1.7	1.1–4.2
Lung – other types	Mineral oil	Any	12	2.0	1.1–3.7
		Long-high	7	4.2	1.8–10.0

[a] Number of exposed cases.
[b] Odds ratio adjusted for many confounders.
CI, confidence interval.

bladder–cutting fluids; kidney–aviation gasoline (which closely resembles unleaded automotive gasoline). To this group of particularly noteworthy associations, it is worth adding one which was generated in an early report based on the first 1487 cases interviewed. It was an analysis of exposure to nickel compounds and we found a significant OR of 3.1 in relation to lung cancer (Gérin et al. 1984). This analysis was not as intensive as those which followed and for that reason we excluded it from the tables in this report.

One general observation is of interest. A disproportionate number of the significant associations concerned lung cancer, either as a whole or some particular histologic subtypes thereof. There are at least three plausible reasons

Table 5. Noteworthy associations between genitourinary cancers and the substances thus far analysed

Site	Substance	Exposure level	n[a]	OR[b]	90% CI
Prostate	Liquid fuels combustion	Any	39	1.7	1.1–2.4
		Long-high	16	2.2	1.2–3.8
Bladder	Synthetic fibers	Any	22	1.8	1.2–2.6
		Long-high	10	2.1	1.1–4.0
Bladder	Cutting fluids	Any	47	1.3	0.9–1.7
		Long-high	15	1.6	0.9–2.6
Bladder	Natural gas combustion	Any	22	1.7	1.1–2.6
		Long-high	10	2.6	1.4–5.0
Kidney	Gasoline exhaust	Any	80	1.2	0.9–1.6
		Long-high	34	1.4	1.0–2.0
Kidney	Aviation gasoline	Any	7	3.1	1.5–6.5
		Long-high	6	3.9	1.7–8.8

[a] Number of exposed cases.
[b] Odds ratio adjusted for many confounders.
CI, confidence interval.

Table 6. Noteworthy associations between lymphomas and the substances thus far analysed

Site	Substance	Exposure level	n[a]	OR[b]	90% CI
Non-Hodgkin's lymphoma	Cotton dust	Any	12	1.5	1.0–2.4
		Long-high	7	3.0	1.5–6.0
Non-Hodgkin's lymphoma	Concrete dust	Any	24	1.2	0.8–1.8
		Long-high	13	2.2	1.3–3.7
Non-Hodgkin's lymphoma	Cutting fluids	Any	22	1.2	0.8–1.8
		Long-high	13	1.8	1.0–3.1
Hodgkin's lymphoma	Mineral spirits	Any	16	1.6	0.8–3.0
		Long-high	12	2.0	1.0–4.1

[a] Number of exposed cases.
[b] Odds ratio adjusted for many confounders.
CI, confidence interval.

for this: (a) The association between lung cancer and cigarette smoking is so strong, and the methods of controlling for confounding imperfect, that there is inevitably some residual confounding when smoking and occupational exposure are associated. (b) The numbers of cases for lung cancer exceeded those for other sites and thus the power to pick up real associations was greater. (c) The lung may be a particularly sensitive target organ for occupational carcinogens. We believe all three of these may have some validity.

Review of Selected Methodologic Findings

Validity of Job History on Interview

The validity of any interview-based case-control study of occupational cancer depends on the accuracy of job histories reported by respondents. For 321 of our study subjects, we carried out a comparison of job histories reported on interview with their corresponding records maintained by the Quebec Pension Plan, a universal government-run pension scheme. The men were interviewed in 1979–1981 about their previous lifetime job history. The Pension Plan had computerized records since 1966 and the comparison between interview and record was carried out on a year by year basis from 1966 through 1978. The record contained only the subject's employer, not his occupation. Thus, what we compared was the employer as reported with the employer as recorded. There was 82% agreement between the record and the interview. Analysis of disagreements showed that these were more likely to be due to the methods of coding employers in the Pension Plan record than to respondent error. We concluded that the validity of job history reports was high (Baumgarten et al. 1983).

Interrater Agreement in Assessment of Exposure

To evaluate the reliability of the exposure assessment process, we undertook six different trials of interrater agreement (Goldberg et al. 1986). Some involved only internal raters from our "in-house" team and others involved comparisons between our internal raters and other external raters who had expertise in certain industries. Ratings were carried out independently by the various participants. In assessing exposure as simply present or absent, two summary indices of agreement were used: per cent with perfect agreement and Cohen's kappa. In most of the trials the per cent with perfect agreement among raters ranged from 95% to 98%, with kappa ranging from 0.5 to 0.7. This relatively high concordance represents a lower limit of our data quality because: (a) these trials were conducted during the first 3 years of our study while the methodology itself was under development and the coders were new to the task, and (b) the trials were carried out among files of workers in particularly complex work environments.

Comparison of Exposure Data Collection Methods for Case-Control Studies

The final part of this presentation concerns the methodology of obtaining occupation exposure information for case-control studies. Our study used a very expensive and time-consuming approach to obtain exposure information. Less expensive approaches have been used such as interview-based studies to obtain and analyse job titles, routine-record based studies (e.g., death certificates) to obtain and analyse job titles and more recently there have been suggestions that job-exposure matrices (JEMs) could provide additional useful information for job title studies.

In the hope of providing guidance as to the relative merits of alternative approaches to exposure data collection in case-control studies of occupation and cancer, we carried out a special series of analyses within our data set (Siemiatycki et al. 1989b). In addition to our own data collection approach, an interview plus a chemist-hygienist evaluation, there were four other strategies which we were able to evaluate: (a) an interview to obtain and analyse job titles only, (b) an interview to obtain job titles supplemented by a JEM applied to the job titles to obtain substance exposures, (c) abstraction of routine records to obtain job titles, and (d) abstraction of job titles from routine records supplemented by a JEM to obtain substance exposures. These are all plausible strategies. The most commonly used ones have been the ones based on job titles only (a and c). The application of a JEM to such data has been widely discussed recently (MRC 1983), but the implementation of such approaches has been hampered by the unavailability of a general purpose good quality JEM. A JEM is simply a method for automatically inferring the job exposures of subjects given their job titles. The five approaches that we compared are listed in Table 7,

Table 7. Main distinguishing features of five types of case-control study design

Design name	Exposure data collection	Exposure variables that can be analysed
REC ONLY	Abstract main job title from routine record	Job titles
REC+JEM	Abstract main job title from routine record	Job titles
	Apply JEM	Substances
INT ONLY	Interview to obtain lifetime job title history	Job titles
INT+JEM	Interview to obtain lifetime job title history	Job titles
	Apply JEM	Substances
INT+CHEM	Interview to obtain detailed lifetime job history	Job titles
	Subject-by-subject exposure assessment	Substances

REC ONLY, routine record only; REC+JEM, REC plus job-exposure matrix; INT ONLY, interview only; INT+JEM, interview plus job-exposure matrix; INT+CHEM, interview plus chemist/hygienist evaluation.

together with the acronym that will be used to designate each one. The objective was to provide a comparison of the relative costs and benefits of the five approaches. Costs were estimated in dollar terms; benefits were estimated in terms of statistical power to detect associations.

Fieldwork costs in epidemiology tend to be very idiosyncratic, depending not only on minutiae of study design but also on the time and place in which the study is carried out and the skill and affiliation of the investigators. Nevertheless, we attempted to roughly cost out the five study designs. We have considered most aspects of the running costs of the study including, where applicable, overhead, case-ascertainment, data abstraction, interviewing, chemical coding, training of chemist-coders, cost of a JEM, and data management. We have excluded some of the most idiosyncratic features like costs of set-up and costs of statistical analysis and reporting. For a study with 500 cases and 500 controls, the expected approximate costs for the five designs would be: INT + CHEM, $450 000; INT + JEM, $170 000; INT ONLY, $150 000; REC + JEM, $50 000; REC ONLY, $30 000. With increasing sample size, the cost of interview-based designs would increase steeply, while costs of routine record-based designs would increase slightly.

Given certain parameters – alpha, sample sizes, relative risk, and prevalence of exposure – there is a well-known method to estimate the statistical power to detect the risk (Schlesselman 1982). If there is nondifferential misclassification error in the attribution of exposure, then this will reduce the relative risk estimate and in turn reduce the statistical power. In fact, if the degree of misclassification can be quantified, then the formula for computing power can be adapted to estimate statistical power in the presence of misclassification. In comparing designs what we are comparing is different degrees of validity of exposure assessment. This can be expressed in terms of sensitivity and specificity. If we know the sensitivity and specificity of one design as compared with another, which might be considered the standard, then we can compute the power of the alternative design vis-à-vis that of the standard. We adopted design INT + CHEM as the standard and computed power of the others relative to this one. The loss in power of different approaches was computed in two stages. First, we estimated the sensitivity and specificity of exposure data generated by each design using as the "gold standard" the information available from design INT + CHEM. Then we applied an algorithm, which allowed us to compute the power when the exposure variable was measured with a certain specified sensitivity and specificity (Siemiatycki et al. 1989b).

Statistical power was computed for the situation where the relative risk as measured in design INT + CHEM = 2.0, alpha = 0.05, and number of cases = number of controls = 500.

Our own ongoing study involved interviews to obtain lifetime job histories of 4261 men, who had a total of nearly 15 000 jobs. For each job our team of chemists had determined whether there was exposure to each of 300 different substances on a checklist. The prevalence of exposure to these substances, along with the above assumptions (i.e., risk ratio (RR) = 2.0; alpha = 0.05, $N = 2 \times 500$)

allowed the computation of statistical power corresponding to each substance in the INT+CHEM design. We limited the study to the 160 most prevalent substances in our data bank.

To compute the power of the other four designs a number of devices were used. To evaluate the INT+JEM design, it was necessary to create a JEM. This was based on the empirical matrix with entries indicating the proportion of men in job i who were considered exposed to substance j. For each of the 160 substances we applied the derived matrix to our data bank of 4261 job histories. This generated an exposure status for each person which could be cross-tabulated with his exposure status as given by the chemists, i.e., the "gold standard." It was thus possible to derive a 2×2 table for exposure to substance j as given by the chemist and by the job title plus JEM, and thereby to derive the sensitivity and specificity of the INT+JEM design. With the derived sensitivity and specificity it was possible to derive the resultant statistical power. This was repeated for each of the 160 substances evaluated, and we thus derived the distribution of power.

A substance-cancer association detectable in the INT+CHEM design might also be detectable by analysing a job title-cancer association. That is, the substance may be strongly enough correlated with a particular occupation that the job title-cancer analysis picks up the corresponding substance-cancer association.

In order to estimate the power of the INT ONLY strategy to pick up the 160 associations under consideration, we examined for each substance that job code which was most strongly correlated with the substance, using the job code histories obtained in the interview. This job code was then used as a surrogate measure for exposure to the substance. This again led to a 2×2 table allowing the estimation of sensitivity and specificity when the optimal job code is used as a surrogate for exposure to the substance. And thus we computed the corresponding power. This was repeated for all 160 substances and provided the distribution of power according to this surrogate.

Our study involved interviews with subjects to obtain lifetime job histories. There was no routine record abstraction of job information. However, for the purpose of evaluating the REC+JEM and REC ONLY designs, we carried out a special data collection.

Medical records of all interviewed patients were reviewed and job information was abstracted. For the evaluation of the REC+JEM and REC ONLY designs, we included only those subjects with mention of occupation in the record. With the job codes abstracted we proceeded to estimate power for REC+JEM in a fashion analogous to that used for INT+JEM (the same JEM was used) and for REC ONLY in an analogous fashion to that used for INT ONLY.

Table 8 summarizes the statistical power to detect a given risk in the five strategies. By definition, the INT+CHEM strategy, the gold standard, provides greatest power. Power is lost in other strategies because the twofold risk that is assumed in the INT+CHEM strategy is diluted by misclassification, and the

Table 8. Distribution of the power to detect substance-cancer associations for each design based on 160 substances

	Power[a]					
Design	0.05–0.19	0.20–0.39	0.40–0.59	0.60–0.79	0.80–1.0	Total
REC ONLY	153	7	0	0	0	160
REC+JEM	51	92	15	2	0	160
INT ONLY	23	95	38	4	0	160
INT+JEM	12	33	54	31	30	160
INT+CHEM	0	0	8	9	143	160

[a] Power to detect twofold risk with alpha = 0.05 and $n = 2 \times 500$. The twofold risk is that obtained in the INT + CHEM design. For the other designs, misclassification leads to a lower relative risk that must be detected, and thereby lower power.
Note that with an alpha level of 0.05, the lower limit of power is also 0.05. For abbreviations, see Table 7.

other strategies are therefore required to detect relative risks lower than 2. As the relative risk to be detected decreases, for fixed sample size and alpha, the power decreases.

The REC ONLY strategy provides hopelessly low power. The INT ONLY strategy is rather better, with 42 of the 160 substances being detectable with greater than 0.40 power. The use of our JEM significantly improves the power of the data bases, and in particular the INT + JEM strategy retains reasonably high power (i.e., > 0.60) for 61 of the 160 substances.

The above results on power are anchored in the particular 160 substances chosen for study and their distribution across job categories. For these and similar substances, the power to pick up a twofold risk using a job code analysis – either INT ONLY or REC ONLY – would be very low. The only way that a job code analysis could be expected to detect a risk would be: if the risk due to the substance were much greater than twofold, or if the sample sizes were much greater than 500, or if the carcinogenic risk factor was very strong in a particular occupation.

In a typical population-based case-control study, there are very few occupations to which a large percentage of men have been exposed. In our study population, using the four-digit level of the Canadian Classification and Dictionary of Occupations (1974), most of the job titles had between 0.1% and 1.0% lifetime prevalence. Only 13 four-digit job codes had greater than 5% lifetime prevalence as compared with 103 substances which had greater than 5% lifetime prevalence. The lower prevalence of job titles as compared with substances mitigates against the usefulness of the former in population-based case-control studies.

Conclusions

The study design we have been using is very expensive compared with other conceivable designs for case-control studies. The data collected in this design are probably of better quality than can be obtained using other approaches. It is not evident whether the benefit to be derived is worth the extra expense. If a good quality JEM were available, then the application of the JEM to job codes obtained by interview or even by routine record abstraction would allow some associations to be detected. If necessary, statistical power could be improved by increasing sample size; this is particularly feasible in the context of a routine record study. However, at present there is no generally available good quality JEM. We hope to develop one. In the absence of a JEM, investigators analyse job titles. Statistical power to detect risk is generally very low with such data.

The case-control study undertaken in Montreal in 1979 has begun providing substantive results. These are in our view important results to follow up and to compare with those of other investigators. It is too soon to be able to evaluate the absolute cost-effectiveness of the expensive approach we took. In the fullness of time, it will be seen whether the evidence produced by our study, both the "positive" and "negative" evidence, is valid and indicative.

References

Baumgarten M, Siemiatycki J, Gibbs GW (1983) Validity of work histories obtained by interview for epidemiologic purposes. Am J Epidemiol 118: 583–591

Canadian Classification and Dictionary of Occupations (1974) Vol I. Manpower and Immigration Canada. Information Canada, Montreal

Doll R, Peto R (1981) The causes of cancer: quantitative estimates of avoidable risks of cancer in the United States today. JNCI 66: 1191–1308

Gérin M, Siemiatycki J, Richardson L, Pellerin J, Lakhani R, Dewar R (1984) Nickel and cancer associations from a multicancer occupation exposure case-referent study: preliminary findings. In: Sunderman FW et al. (eds) Nickel in the human environment, International Agency for Research on Cancer, Lyon (IARC publ no 53)

Gérin M, Siemiatycki J, Kemper H, Bégin D (1985) Obtaining occupation exposure histories in epidemiologic case-control studies. J Occup Med 27: 420–426

Gérin M, Siemiatycki J, Nadon L, Dewar R, Krewski D (1989) Cancer risks due to occupational exposure to formaldehyde: results of a multi-site case-control study in Montreal. Int J Cancer 44: 53–58

Goldberg MS, Siemiatycki J, Gérin M (1986) Inter-rater agreement in assessing occupational exposure in a case-control study. Br J Ind Med 43(10): 667–676

MRC: Medical Research Council (1983) Job exposure matrices. Proceedings of a conference held in April 1982 at the University of Southampton. MRC Environmental Epidemiology Unit, Southampton (Scientific report no 2)

Schlesselman JJ (1982) Case-control studies. Oxford University Press, New York, p 148

Siemiatycki J (1984) An epidemiological approach to discovering occupational carcinogens by obtaining better information on occupational exposures. In: Harring JM (ed)

Recent advances in occupational health, vol 2. Churchill Livingstone, Edinburgh, pp 143–157

Siemiatycki J, Day NE, Fabry J, Cooper JA (1981) Discovering carcinogens in the occupational environment: a novel epidemiologic approach. JNCI 66: 217–225

Siemiatycki J, Richardson L, Gérin M, Goldberg M, Dewar R, Désy M, Campbell S, Wacholder S (1986) Associations between several sites of cancer and nine organic dusts: results from an hypothesis-generating case-control study in Montreal, 1979–83. Am J Epidemiol 123(2): 235–249

Siemiatycki J, Dewar R, Nadon L, Gérin M, Richardson L, Wacholder S (1987a) Associations between several sites of cancer and twelve petroleum-derived liquids: results from a case-control study in Montreal. Scand J Work Environ Health 13: 493–504

Siemiatycki J, Wacholder S, Richardson L, Dewar R, Gérin M (1987b) Discovering carcinogens in the occupational environment: method of data collection and analysis of a large case-referent monitoring system. Scand J Work Environ Health 13: 486–492

Siemiatycki J, Gérin M, Stewart P, Nadon L, Dewar R, Richardson L (1988) Associations between several sites of cancer and ten types of exhaust and combustion products: results from a case-referent study in Montreal. Scand J Work Environ Health 14: 79–90

Siemiatycki J, Dewar R, Lakhani R, Nadon L, Richardson L, Gérin M (1989a) Cancer risks associated with ten inorganic dusts: results from a case-control study in Montreal. Am J Industr Med 16: 547–567

Siemiatycki J, Dewar R, Richardson L (1989b) Costs and statistical power associated with five methods of collecting occupation exposure information for population-based case-control studies. Am J Epidemiol 130(6): 1236–1246

Thomas DC, Siemiatycki J, Dewar R, Robins J, Goldberg M, Armstrong B (1985) The problem of multiple inference in studies designed to generate hypotheses. Am J Epidemiol 122(6): 1080–1095

Recent Approaches to Retrospective Exposure Assessment in Occupational Cancer Epidemiology

M. Gérin

Département de Médecine du Travail et d'Hygiène du Milieu, Faculté de Médecine, Université de Montréal, C.P. 6128, Succursale A, Montréal, Québec H3C 3J7, Canada

Introduction

The primary aim in occupational cancer epidemiology is the identification of carcinogens, thus allowing the implementation of preventive measures. The identification of carcinogens rests on the retrospective assessment of subjects' specific occupational exposures, beyond the basic assessment of their occupational titles. Various efforts have resulted in standardized methods for disease assessment and sophistication in various aspects of study design and statistical methods. It is, however, becoming recognized that too little emphasis has been placed on the crucial exposure variable in the exposure-disease tandem. Indeed retrospective assessment of exposure to specific chemical agents is fraught with several difficulties related to, inter alia, (a) the obtaining of subjects' occupational histories with detailed and relevant information; (b) the complexity of most workplace environments with exposures being to mixtures of agents as a rule rather than as an exception; and (c) the lack of systematic industrial hygiene documentation on past and even present levels of exposure for most industries and occupations and for the majority of chemical agents.

The various approaches to retrospective exposure assessment that have been developed over the years depend on a number of critical factors such as (a) the basic design of the study, being either population based or cohort based (including case-control studies within a cohort); (b) the level of detail on occupational history with, at one extreme death certificate information on last occupation held and, at the other, a complete face-to-face interview with the subject with the use of relevant questionnaires; (c) the nature of the chemical exposure(s) investigated, being either easily recognizable or well-documented substances such as wood or asbestos dust, or agents necessitating a more complex assessment procedure such as formaldehyde or a given specific solvent; and (d) the number of agents investigated, being either limited to one or a few in most hypothesis-testing types of studies and studies aiming at estimating etiological fractions, or potentially large in hypothesis-generating studies.

It is the purpose of this report to review methods in the field of retrospective exposure assessment, and more specifically on recent developments for population-based studies. The job-exposure matrix (JEM) approach and the use

Recent Results in Cancer Research, Vol. 120

of expert coders in the framework of a large hypothesis-generating case-control study in Montreal are described by way of illustration. Emphasis has been put on the "mechanics" of exposure assessment rather than on the epidemiological uses or advantages of the various methods.

Retrospective Exposure Assessment in Cohort Studies

One of the most classical type of studies is the retrospective cohort study where the mortality or morbidity experience of a group of workers having worked in the past for a company or in a specific industry is compared with that of a suitable reference group. Cohorts may equally be defined on the basis of a specific profession or occupation which could regroup several employers. In cohort studies exposure is often simply defined as having worked for a minimum given amount of time in the company, industry or occupation under investigation. When more specific information is available, various subclassification schemes can be adopted to regroup workers into various separate exposure subgroups i.e. by administrative category (clerical, maintenance, operations, laboratory), by geographical subdivision (specific buildings, plants or departments), by occupational title related to process and task, or by a combination of these approaches (Esmen 1979; Gamble and Spirtas 1976; Nelson et al. 1983).

The cohort study may provide the ideal situation, however, for assessment of exposure to specific agents. This usually involves a limited number of exposures and job situations and potential availability of detailed retrospective information on processes and agents. Even though exposure assessment has often been limited to a judgement on the presence or absence of exposure, several schemes have been used whereby exposure has been evaluated on a semiquantitative scale such as low-medium-high or more detailed yet qualitative indices taking into account such elements as proximity to the source of exposure, time spent exposed, possibility of spikes or spills, or of cutaneous contact (Bend et al. 1986; Greenberg and Tamburro 1981).

In several instances, however, it has been possible to associate quantitative levels of exposure to the subjects' various job titles or work situations. These are usually best estimates based on a combination of the following sources of information: past and present industrial hygiene measurements; company files on processes; interviews with engineers, foremen and workers about past conditions and their integration into exposure assessment panels; and even physical reconstitution of past conditions (Armstrong et al. 1986; Steward et al. 1986). In those situations where information, either qualitative or quantitative, on exposure to a series of agents has been systematically evaluated over all job titles within a cohort, one can conveniently refer to the set of data as a JEM. In contrast to JEMs developed in the population-based study context (see below) these matrices are usually too idiosyncratic to be directly usable outside of their own cohort.

Exposure Assessment in Population-Based Studies

In population-based studies, where by definition subjects' jobs cover a very broad spectrum of occupations and industries, it is usually impractical or impossible to access exposure information directly from individual employers. Indeed the only exposure information available is often limited to the subjects' main job titles. This is the case, for instance, in many large death certificate- or register-based surveillance or case-control studies. When basic information on exposure is limited to job titles it may be possible to generate specific exposure information through the use of a job exposure matrix; this methodology is presented in a subsequent section.

In studies based on questionnaires, specific questions may be asked on use or exposure to the agents of interest and the subjects' answers used directly as evidence. This self-report approach has the obvious advantage of simplicity and can be easily implemented for a number of common agents or general categories of exposures that can be validly reported by a general population e.g. wood dust or cutting oils or gasoline. Its validity is highly questionable, however, for the majority of individual chemicals, whose names or presence in the work environment are usually unknown to the working population, e.g. formaldehyde or benzene. Self-report may furthermore be tainted by the phenomenon of differential recall between cases and controls. Means have been proposed in order to evaluate the importance of this recall bias in a given study (Axelson 1980).

Another approach to specific exposure assessment is through interpretation of the available information on each subject's work history. In the usual hypothesis-testing situation this may simply involve the traditional regrouping of subjects on the basis of job titles that are judged to bring out exposure to a common agent. If, however, detailed job descriptions have been obtained through the use of a work history questionnaire, it may be possible to infer potential exposure to the investigated agents by using such expertise as that of industrial hygienists (Hernberg et al. 1983). This task may be facilitated if specialized questionnaires have been used that are specifically designed to elicit critical information on the agents of interest. The use of exposure assessment experts in the framework of a large occupational cancer hypothesis-generating case-control study in Montreal is detailed in a subsequent section.

Job-Exposure Matrices in Population-Based Studies

A JEM is basically "an occupation and exposure linkage system" (Hoar et al. 1980), systematically documenting a number of exposures over the complete range of occupations encountered in the general population. Practically speaking it is a data bank characterized by the following elements: (a) a job classification consisting of either a classification of occupational titles or industrial (economic) activities, or a cross-classification integrating both dimensions; (b) a list of agents of interest; and (c) an indication for each combination of job and agent on whether and to what extent exposure takes place, using a given index of exposure.

These exposure values, constituting the core of the matrix, are assigned by taking into account one or several potential sources of information based on bibliographical data, consultation with experts or industrial hygiene surveys. Table 1 summarizes the main features of matrices for which published descriptions are available. The development of JEMs can be seen to be still quite limited with basically four groups of investigators from three countries having been involved. The matrix from Hoar et al. (1980) served as a pioneering work, opening the way for the U.K. matrix from Pannett et al. (1985) and the Italian matrices (Macaluso et al. 1983; Vineis and Magnani 1985) developed by closely collaborating investigators. It can readily be seen from Table 1 that the matrices presented differ considerably in their main features, i.e., the job classifications used and the ways to combine them, the number and the nature of the agents included, the indices of exposure, as well as the sources of information used.

Except in the case of the NIOSH matrix, based on a walk-through survey of a sample of U.S. industries, exposure values are essentially judgemental, reflecting the best evaluations of a small group of experts from nonsystematically organized sources of information. (The NIOSH matrix itself is not based on actual measurements of agents but on their observation in workplaces.) The validity of JEM data can further be questioned in relation to the known variations of exposure patterns in time (from era to era) and in space (in different regions or countries). More generally, exposure misclassification in matrices results from the fact that job titles are usually not precise enough in terms of actual tasks performed or processes used, thus diluting exposures specifically encountered by subgroups. This type of error results in biasing exposure-disease associations towards null.

Except in the case of the prototype matrix of Hoar et al., other population-based matrices have as yet been the object of little usage by groups other than their originators. This may be explained partly by the anticipated pitfalls of the method, already alluded to, but also by the relative recency of their introduction. Even though the most obvious potential epidemiological applications of JEMs are to studies where subjects' exposure information is limited to job titles, they may additionally find use as a complement or basis to other types of exposure assessment such as subject by subject expert judgements.

Clearly more work is necessary, such as the completion of studies using presently available matrices, to fully evaluate this strategy of exposure assessment. The introduction of more objective matrices, derived from survey data, such as the NIOSH matrix, holds great promise. New matrices may also fruitfully develop from the set of exposure data collected in the framework of large case-control studies with subject by subject exposure assessment performed by experts (Gérin et al. 1985).

Table 1. Main features of five population-based job exposure matrices

Origin	Job classification	Agents	Index of exposure	Sources of information
Hoar et al. (1980) U.S.	ca. 500 categories (combined U.S. industrial and occupational titles classifications)	ca. 400 toxic chemical agents + radiations	Low, moderate, high[a]	Literature
Pannett et al. (1985) U.K.	669 categories (combined U.K. classifications of occupations and industries)	49 agents, chemical and physical	Low, moderate, high[b]	Literature, experts
Vineis and Magnani (1985) Turin, Italy	ILO occupational titles and U.N. industry classification (separate)	74 chemical agents (carcinogens)	absent/present	Literature, experts
Macaluso et al. (1983) Milan, Italy	Same as Vineis and Magnani (1985), above[c]	8 lung carcinogens	4 degrees[d]	Literature, experts
K. Sieber, personal communication, NIOSH, U.S.	U.S. industrial and occupational title classifications (occupations nested within industries)	8342 hazards (chemical, physical, biological)	Proportion exposed	U.S. National Occupational Hazard survey

[a] According to degree of hazard and some judgemental evaluation.
[b] Based on a combination of proportion of workforce exposed and extent of exposure.
[c] Only job industry titles corresponding to subjects in a Milan lung cancer study are included.
[d] According to both level of exposure and probability of exposure above general population levels.

Subject by Subject Exposure Assessment by Experts in a Large Population-Based Case-Control Study in Montreal

Since 1979, a large case-control study of occupational cancer has been under way in Montreal. Only methods of exposure assessment are summarized here, as an example of what could be achieved in population-based hypothesis-generating studies where experts are asked to evaluate a multiplicity of exposures from questionnaire data. Details of the study design, general methods and some results can be found in a number of reports (Gérin et al. 1984, 1985; Goldberg et al. 1986; Siemiatycki et al. 1981, 1986, 1987a, b, 1988). About 20 sites of cancer were selected for study. The target population consisted of males aged 35–70 years, resident in the area of Montreal. Cases eligible were incident from 1979 to 1985. Altogether ca. 4600 cases were ascertained and, for 3700, interviews (92%) or self-administered questionnaires (8%) were obtained. The primary strategy has been to compare each case series with a control group drawn from among the other sites.

The Occupational Interview

A group of trained interviewers were involved in the critical step of administering the questionnaire to each subject as soon as he was identified. Occupational history is obtained through the use of a semistructured general questionnaire covering, for each job of each subject, the following points: (a) activity of employer or company, (b) occupation of subject, (c) description of specific tasks, machines and materials used, and (d) description of the work environment in terms of the usual place of work, the presence of dusts, fumes, gases or vapours, the activities of other workers and the use of protective equipment. Most of the questions are open-ended with the subject being encouraged to give as much detail as possible on his work activities and conditions. Having realized early that exposure assessment would be rendered easier if some specialized questions were asked in order to probe specific professions, a set of profession-specific questionnaires have been developed (e.g. welders, painters). These are administered immediately after the general occupational questionnaire.

Interviewers and hygienist-coders have ample opportunity to interact with each other in order to discuss interviewing problems, improve the technical proficiency of interviewers and the acceptability of specialized questionnaires.

Translating Occupational Histories into Exposure Histories

A team of three to four chemists and hygienists has been given the task of exposure assessment. A brief outline of the developed methodology is presented.

A coding checklist of some 275 occupational exposures of sufficient prevalence and well-documented in the literature has been established. These agents include some specific chemicals (e.g. benzene), chemical groups or functions (e.g., aromatic amines), mixtures of relatively fixed composition (e.g. gasoline) or variable composition (e.g. paints), complex materials (e.g. cement), as well as general categories (e.g. solvents). A few radiations are also included. The complete list of agents is given in Appendix 1 of the report by Gérin et al. (1985). Agents are classified into categories according to their usual physical state: dusts, gases, fumes and smoke, liquids and their vapours, and a special category for chemical groups. To each possible exposure of a worker, coders associate the following qualitative indices of exposure: (a) reliability, indicating the coder's estimate of the degree of certainty that the worker has been occupationally exposed to the substance (1, possible; 2, probable; 3, certain); (b) level, indicating the relative average level of exposure to the substance according to a scale specific to each agent (1, low; 2, medium; 3, high); and (c) frequency, indicating the average proportion of working time during which exposure occurred at the level coded (1, less than 5% of time; 2, from 5% to 30%; and 3, more than 30%). Additionally, a contact code indicates whether exposure was respiratory, cutaneous or both. Coders are experienced chemists or hygienists. They complement their own knowledge with information provided by the scientific and technical literature, trade directories and frequent contact with experts or consultants from industry or the occupational safety and health network. Each occupational history is examined successively by at least three coders with the objective of deriving a consensus coding.

Exposure Assessment Validity

The exposure coding method presented relies largely on the judgement of the chemist-coders. In order to shed light on the accuracy of their assessments several trials of inter-rater agreement were implemented (Goldberg et al. 1986). Some of these trials involved only internal raters, whereas others involved comparisons between the internal raters and other external raters who had expertise in certain industries. The six trials involved a limited number of job descriptions with the following characteristics: paint industry (inside and outside raters), rubber industry (inside raters), welding activities (inside and outside raters), chemical manufacturing (inside and outside raters), metal products manufacturing (inside and outside raters) and a miscellaneous assortment (code-recode by internal raters).

In assessing exposure as simply present or absent, two summary indices of agreement were used: per cent with perfect agreement and Cohen's kappa. In most of the trials the per cent with perfect agreement among raters ranged from 95% to 98%, with kappa ranging from 0.5 to 0.7. The kappas were slightly higher for internal-internal comparisons than for internal-external ones. These results indicate a relatively high degree of inter-rater agreement over a range of industries, occupations and time periods of employment.

Even though these results lend credibility to the overall validity of this type of retrospective exposure assessment, there is little data in the literature to allow comparisons to be made. Furthermore, the degree of agreement from substance to substance has not been evaluated in these trials. More work is in progress to clarify this last point.

Discussion

After 8 years of involvement in the development and implementation of a particular type of exposure assessment method, several comments may be ventured that could perhaps be useful to other investigators. For the most part these remarks are relevant to the situation of a population-based hypothesis-generating case-control study, though they may also be relevant to other designs such as cohort or nested case-control studies or job-title based studies making use of JEMs.

Feasibility

Our experience is ample evidence that implementing a wide range exposure assessment method is feasible. The financial aspects and merits of this type of study are presented in a companion report (Siemiatycki et al., this volume). It is also clear that, because of the innovative nature of this assignment, a long developmental period has preceded the full-scale implementation period. It can be expected that, in any study of this type, extensive time will be allocated, inter alia, to hiring and training of chemists and hygienists, to the establishment of an extensive and systematically organized literature data bank on exposures, jobs and industries and to the set-up of basic exposure profiles to be used as a basis for exposure coding.

Possible improvement in the exposure assessment process would be through the use of an integrated computerized information management system through which chemists could have direct screen access to all job descriptions and previous codings, with word searching features, the capability of sorting files by occupational and industry titles, company names and years. Access to exposure data banks such as existing JEMs and industrial hygiene data bases could be an additional feature.

Importance of Questionnaire and Interviewers

The exposure assessment step is strongly dependent on the quality of the information provided to the coders by the interviewers. In our type of hypothesis-generating study we had to use a semistructured type of questionnaire with no specific emphasis on certain types of exposure. We found, however, that a set of questions directed towards specific professions (specialized questionnaires) could greatly improve the reliability and ease of coding.

This strategy could be fully developed by implementing specific questionnaires covering systematically all potentially exposed job situations.

Answers to open-ended questionnaires such as were used in this study are dependent on the proficiency of the interviewer both in technical matters and in his/her human approach towards the subject. Furthermore, chemists have noted shifts in the quality of interviews over time. This has been attributed to a kind of burnout of interviewers who are faced with a more demanding job than in the case of a structured questionnaires. One last point worth noting is that the quality of coding was found to be better when chemists were dealing with interviewer administered questionnaires than with self-administered questionnaires. The latter had to be used for 8% of the subjects who could not be interviewed.

Limits on Number and Type of Exposures

Even though tens of thousands of different specific chemicals may find their way into the work environment only a small fraction of these may reasonably be coded in such a type of study. The main criteria that limit the number and type of exposures that can be assessed are (a) the prevalence of the agents, even though this criterion is partly a function of the sample size expected and (b) the presence and the quality of documentation on agents. As a result only the most frequent exposures and those having been the object of previous occupational studies can be assessed the most reliably. The length of our coding list (of some 275 agents) represents, we believe, an upper limit to what can be routinely assessed. It is worth noting that a high proportion of agents on our list represent mixtures, broad categories of products or chemical families.

Indices of Exposure

In the course of this project we have developed and consistently used three main indices to describe exposure, namely level, frequency and reliability. All three indices are on a three-point scale (low, medium, high, plus the implicit zero for not coded). The relative and qualitative nature of these indices needs to be stressed, however. For instance, generally, it is impossible to formally assign concentration ranges to the various level points. It is important, however, to attempt to associate, as reference categories, typical jobs to the various index values for each agent. We are satisfied with these types of indices which have provided the necessary flexibility for exposure judgement. Furthermore, in the analysis, the statistician has the opportunity to combine these indices in various ways. Other approaches to the definition of exposure indices may be equally appropriate.

Conclusions

Most of the main methods of exposure assessment in occupational cancer epidemiology have been reviewed in this report with varying levels of detail. It is rather clear that there is no standardized method applicable to all studies but rather a strong dependence on the basic epidemiological design of each study (population- or cohort-based, hypothesis-testing or -generating) and on idiosyncratic factors such as financial resources and ease of access to information sources.

Some common important features of methods of specific exposure assessment can be summarized as the following conclusions or recommendations: (a) emphasis to be placed on the front-end of the studies i.e. questionnaires and interviewers; (b) involvement of exposure specialists, mainly industrial hygienists or chemists but also engineers, foremen and workers; (c) the need to characterize exposure by precisely defining the agents and indices of exposure; (d) the need to validate the exposure assessment process by implementing, when feasible, comparison trials or by pulling expertise from various sources; and (e) the need to develop new tools such as industrial hygiene data bases and job-exposure matrices.

References

Armstrong BG, Tremblay CG, Cyr D, Theriault GP (1986) Estimating the relationship between exposure to tar volatiles and the incidence of bladder cancer in aluminum smelter workers. Scand J Work Environ Health 12: 486–493

Axelson O (1980) A note on observational bias in case-referent studies in occupational health epidemiology. Scand J Work Environ Health 6: 80–82

Bend GG, Flores GH, Shellenberger RJ, Cartmill JB, Fishbeck WA, Cook RR (1986) Nested case-control study of lung cancer among chemical workers. Am J Epidemiol 124: 53–66

Esmen N (1979) Retrospective industrial hygiene surveys. Am Ind Hyg Assoc J 40: 58–65

Gamble J, Spirtas R (1976) Job Classification and utilization of complete work histories in occupational epidemiology. J Occup Med 18: 399–404

Gérin M, Siemiatycki J, Richardson L, Pellerin J, Lakhani R, Dewar R (1984) Nickel and cancer associations from a multicancer occupation exposure case-referent study: preliminary findings. In: Sunderman F (ed) Nickel in the environment. International Agency for Research on Cancer, Lyon, pp 105–115

Gérin M, Siemiatycki J, Kemper H, Begin D (1985) Obtaining occupation exposure histories in epidemiologic case-control studies. J Occup Med 27: 420–426

Goldberg M, Siemiatycki J, Gérin M (1986) Inter-rater agreement in assessing occupational exposure in case-control study. Br J Ind Med 43: 667–676

Greenberg RA, Tamburro CH (1981) Exposure indices for epidemiological surveillance of carcinogenic agents in an industrial chemical environment. J Occup Med 23: 353–358

Hernberg S, Westerholm P, Schultz-Larsen K, Degerth R, Kuosma E, Englund A, Engzell U, Sand Hansen H, Mutanen P (1983) Nasal and sinonasal cancer. Connection with occupational exposures in Denmark, Finland and Sweden. Scand J Work Environ Health 9: 315–326

Hoar SK, Morrison AS, Cole P, Silverman DT (1980) An occupation and exposure linkage system for the study of occupational carcinogenesis. J Occup Med 22: 722–726

Macaluso M, Vineis P, Continenza D, Ferrario F, Pisani P, Andisio R (1983) Job exposure matrices: experience in Italy. In: Job exposure matrices. Medical Research Council, Southampton, pp 22–30 (Scientific report no 2)

Nelson NA, Barker DM, Van Peena PFD, Blanchard AG (1983) Determining exposure categories for a refinery retrospective cohort mortality study. Am Ind Hyg Assoc J 46: 653–657

Pannett B, Coggon D, Acheson ED (1985) A job-exposure matrix for use in population-based studies in England and Wales. Br J Ind Med 42: 777–783

Siemiatycki J, Day N, Fabry J, Cooper J (1981) Discovering carcinogens in the occupational environment: a novel epidemiologic approach. J NCI 66: 217–225

Siemiatycki J, Richardson J, Gérin M, Goldberg M, Dewar R, Desy M, Campbell S, Wacholder S (1986) Associations between several sites of cancer and nine organic dusts: results from an hypothesis-generating case-control study in Montreal 1979–83. Am J Epidemiol 123: 235–249

Siemiatycki J, Dewar R, Nadon L, Gérin M, Richardson L, Wacholder S (1987a) Associations between several sites of cancer and 12 petroleum-derived liquids: results from a case-control study in Montreal. Scand J Work Environ Health 13: 493–504

Siemiatycki J, Wacholder S, Richardson L, Dewar R, Gérin M (1987b) Discovering carcinogens in the occupational environment: methods of data collection and analysis of a large case-control monitoring system. Scand J Work Environ Health 13: 486–492

Siemiatycki J, Gérin M, Stewart P, Nadon L, Dewar R, Richardson L (1988) Associations between several sites of cancer and ten types of exhaust and combustion products: results from a case-referent study in Montreal. Scand J Work Environ Health 14: 79–90

Steward PA, Blair A, Cubit DA, Bales RE, Kaplan SA, Ward J, Goffey W, O'Berg M, Walrath J (1986) Estimating historical exposure to formaldehyde in a retrospective mortality study. Appl Ind Hyg 1: 34–41

Vineis P, Magnani C (1985) Occupation and bladder cancer in males: a case-control study. Int J Cancer 35: 599–606

*Effects of Measurement Errors on Estimates of Exposure-Response Relationships**

B. Armstrong

McGill University, School of Occupational Health, 1130 Pine Avenue West, Montreal, Quebec H3A 1A3, Canada

Introduction

Establishing a causal association between an occupational exposure and the incidence of cancer requires the consideration of many criteria. One of these is whether an association between level of exposure and risk has been demonstrated. For this purpose an association between an ordinal measure of exposure (e.g. three exposure categories) and risk is generally considered sufficient. Once a causal association has been established with reasonable certainty, interest often focusses on a more quantitative relationship between an absolute measure of exposure and risk – for a given quantity of exposure, what is the increase in risk? In particular, estimates of such relationships are required to inform the process of setting standards for "acceptable" limits of exposure. This paper is relevant mainly to these quantitative estimates of exposure-response relationships.

All estimates of exposure-response relationships made from epidemiological studies require estimates of exposure for persons in the study. However exposure is measured, there is almost always a possibility of error. We are concerned here with exposures measured on a numerical scale. In this case, the amount by which the measurement differs from the "true" exposure (often hypothetical), is called measurement error. The notion of true exposure here is not absolute (such as a biologically effective dose), but relative. Usually it will represent the exposure that would have been observed had the worker worn an accurate personal dosimeter throughout their working life. The error may be systematic (constant for all persons in the study) or random, or a combination of both. We can generally work out the effect of systematic measurement error on estimates of exposure-response relationships from common-sense arguments. The effect of random measurement error can be more obscure. The objective of this paper is to provide an overview, accessible to epidemiologists, of the basic statistical results relevant in the context of occupational cancer epidemiology. A general epidemiological review in the context of dietary studies is given by Willett

* Supported by a grant from the Institut de recherche en santé et sécurité au travail.

Recent Results in Cancer Research, Vol. 120

(1989). Throughout, emphasis is on simple results, which are obtained by making assumptions which may not be well approximated in all situations.

Attenuation Due to Measurement Error in Simple Linear Regression

Defining x as true exposure and z as the (approximate) measurement of x, we may write:

$$z = x + e \tag{1}$$

where e is an additive measurement error. In the usual ("classical") measurement error model we assume error e to have a distribution independent of the true value x, with no systematic error, so that the average z of many replicated measurements $z_1, z_2, \ldots$ of the same x is x, i.e. $E(e|x)=0$ and $E(z|x)=x$. Measurement error e does not depend on outcome y in this model (i.e. it is "nondifferential"). We shall also assume for simplicity that the distributions of error e and true exposures x are normal (Gaussian), although most of results below (but less so in the third section) are valid more generally.

In the simple linear regression model a response y measured on a numerical scale depends on true x according to the regression equation:

$$y = \beta_0 + \beta_1 x + \varepsilon, \tag{2}$$

where ε is a random variable with zero mean, here taken to be normally distributed. Although response is rarely measured on a numerical scale in cancer epidemiology, we consider this model first because of its simplicity, and the generalizability of many results obtained for it.

The relationship between y and the approximate exposure z is:

$$y = \beta_0^* + \beta_1^* z + \varepsilon^* \tag{3}$$

with β_0^* and β_1^* not equal to β_0 and β_1. In particular

$$\beta_1^* = R\beta_1, \tag{4}$$

where R is the reliability of z as a measurement of x, equal to the proportion of variance of z which is due to x, i.e.

$$R = \mathrm{var}(x)/\mathrm{var}(z) = \mathrm{var}(x)/\{\mathrm{var}(x) + \mathrm{var}(e)\}. \tag{5}$$

Equivalently R is the square of the correlation of x and z. Since $0 < R < 1$ the regression line is made less steep (attenuated) by random measurement error. The overall effect of measurement error is to tilt the regression line about a fulcrum at the point $(\mu_y, \mu_z) = (\mu_y, \mu_x)$, where μ_y, μ_x, and μ_z are the mean response, true, and observed exposures in the study population.

If R is known, an unbiased ("corrected for attenuation" or "deattenuated") estimate of the true slope β_1, is obtainable from a "naive" estimate $\hat{\beta}_1^*$ using approximate exposures, as $\hat{\beta}_1 = \hat{\beta}_1^*/R$. Valid confidence intervals for β_1 may be constructed (from those for β_1^*) by applying the correction factor $(1/R)$ to the limits obtained for β_1^* by the usual methods. The estimation of R from available validity or reliability data sets is discussed below.

The usual t-test and F-test against the null hypothesis that $\beta_1^* = 0$, carried out using the approximate data $\{y, z\}$, are also valid tests against the same hypothesis for the true parameter $\beta_1 = 0$; i.e. for testing we can ignore measurement error. Furthermore, this "naive" test is as powerful as possible given that the data were measured with error, although such a test will have less power than one based on the data without such error.

The basic results for measurement error in linear regression have been known for many years, and details are presented in some elementary statistics textbooks (e.g. Snedecor and Cochran 1967). Cochran (1968) summarizes many useful results, and Fuller (1987) includes an authoritative discussion and review of this and other models in which y is measured on a numerical scale.

Attenuation Due to Measurement Error in Relative Risk Regression

The Relative Risk Regression Model

In cancer epidemiology, where interest is in the effect of exposure on disease incidence, or equivalently survival (time to disease occurrence), simple regression for a numerical response is not appropriate. However, regression models for relative risks have become increasingly popular in this context (see Prentice and Farewell 1986 for review). For cohort studies with times of disease occurrence observed, disease rate ratios (here called relative risks) may be regressed on risk factors using "Cox" regression. For case-control studies which are matched or stratified by age, essentially the same relative risk regression model is appropriate.

For a single exposure x, the relative risk model may be written in somewhat simplified form:

$$\mathrm{RR}(x, t) = r\{\beta_1, \mathrm{x}(t)\} \tag{6}$$

Risk in this model is relative to risk at $x=0$, and r is a mathematical function which can take several forms; popular models are the exponential relative risk model (closely related to the logistic model):

$$\mathrm{RR}(x, t) = \exp\{\beta_1 \mathrm{x}(t)\} \tag{7}$$

and the linear relative risk model:

$$\mathrm{RR}(x, t) = 1 + \beta_1 \mathrm{x}(t) \tag{8}$$

The exposure x is written as a function $\mathrm{x}(t)$ of time t (usually age) to stress that the value of x may change with time. A common example in occupational studies is cumulative exposure.

The Effects of Measurement Error

As with simple linear regression, the primary effect of replacing true exposures x with approximate measurements z in the classical measurement error model is to attenuate the regression parameter β_1. Since there is no intercept parameter β_0 the attenuated "naive" regression line is uniformly below the "true" relationship in relative risk regression models (the lines meet at a relative risk of one for zero exposure). Thus, relative risks predicted at given observed approximate levels of exposure are lower than they would be if true risk factor values had been available. For the exponential relative risk model, if measurement error and the true risk factor follow a normal distribution and certain other unexceptional assumptions are met, the attenuation of β_1 is that for β_1 in simple linear regression, i.e. $\beta_1^* = R\beta_1$. Here $R = \text{var}(x)/\{\text{var}(x) + \text{var}(e)\}$ as before, but var(x) is the variance of true exposure *within age strata*. For the linear relative risk model the attenuation is more pronounced:

$$\beta_1^* = [R/\{1 + \beta_1 \mu_x x\ (1 - R)\}]\beta_1 \qquad (9)$$

The extent to which this bias is more severe than that in the exponential model depends on $\beta_1\mu_x$, the mean increment in relative risk in the study population. If var(x) (or μ_x for the linear model) depends strongly on age, these simple formulae become poor approximations. This will be the case if the magnitude of the effects of exposure on mortality is sufficient for early deaths among highly exposed persons to importantly effect the distribution of exposures.

The bias in the relative risk regression parameter β_1 under the exponential and linear models with standard deviation of measurement error (SD(e))

Table 1. Bias in estimated relative risk parameter due to normal measurement error

SD(e)[a] / SD(x)	Exponential model (= R)	Bias in parameter β_1 Linear model with mean relative risk in study population: 1.1	1.5	2.0	5.0
0.00	1.00	1.00	1.00	1.00	1.00
0.10	0.99	0.99	0.99	0.98	0.95
0.20	0.96	0.96	0.94	0.93	0.83
0.30	0.92	0.91	0.88	0.85	0.69
0.40	0.86	0.85	0.81	0.76	0.56
0.50	0.80	0.78	0.73	0.67	0.44
0.75	0.64	0.62	0.54	0.47	0.26
1.00	0.50	0.48	0.40	0.33	0.17
1.50	0.31	0.29	0.23	0.18	0.08
2.00	0.20	0.19	0.14	0.11	0.05

[a] Ratio of standard deviation of errors e to standard deviation of true exposures x.

ranging from 0.1 to 2.0 of a standard deviation of the true exposures (SD(x)) is given in Table 1. (It is this relative variation (SD(e)/SD(x)) which determines R, and hence bias.) Perhaps the most striking observation that we may make from this exercise is that, because reliability R is a ratio of *variances* rather than standard deviations, measurement error with a standard deviation as large as one-half of the standard deviation of the true x results for the exponential relative risk model in an observed regression parameter which is 80% of the true value – a minor bias by most epidemiological standards (Willett 1989). The increase in the degree of bias in β_1 in the linear model relative to the exponential model can be observed to be important only in study populations with quite high mean relative risk. As with simple linear regression, if R is known a corrected estimate and confidence interval (CI) for β_1 in the exponential relative risk model may be obtained by applying the correction factor ($1/R$) to the "naive" estimate $\hat{\beta}_1^*$ and its CI from the observed data z, i.e.

$$\hat{\beta}_1 = \hat{\beta}_1^*/R \tag{10}$$

In the linear model the correction factor is, from (9):

$$\hat{\beta}_1 = \hat{\beta}_1^*/(R - \hat{\beta}_1^* \, \mu_x \, (1 - R)) \tag{11}$$

The "naive" tests against $\beta_1^* = 0$ (e.g. chi-square score, Wald, or likelihood ratio tests) using the crude data are valid and efficient tests for $\beta_1 = 0$, but with less power than those based on true exposures. The efficiency of most types of regression analyses using approximate exposures relative to those using true exposures has been shown in a result of remarkable generality to be equal to reliability R (Lagakos 1987).

Prentice (1982); Armstrong and Oakes (1982); Clayton (1988); Pepe et al. (1989); and Armstrong et al. (1989) discuss measurement error in relative risk models further.

Example

Theriault et al. (1984) and Armstrong et al. (1986) studied the relationship between exposure to coal tar pitch volatiles and bladder cancer in aluminum reduction plant workers. A linear relative risk model of cumulative exposures to benzo-*a*-pyrene (in $\mu g/m^3$ years) fitted the observed data well. The parameter β_1 was estimated at 0.018 (95% CI 0.007–0.042). Table 2 shows the effects of correcting this estimate for measurement error if the normal measurement error model discussed above applied. Effects of mild (SD(e)/SD(x) = 0.1) to quite severe (SD(e)/SD(x) = 0.5) measurement error are shown. To emphasize the practical implication of these corrections, the table also shows the relative risk predicted after 40 years working at 5 $\mu g/m^3$ – the hygiene standard in some countries. At $R = 0.5$ estimates of risk increment become very large, suggesting that the measurement error model assumptions may be unrealistic at these values. Indeed the normal measurement error model is a poor fit to these data

Table 2. Bladder cancer and exposure to coal tar pitch volatiles: estimates of linear relative risk increment corrected for normal measurement error

$\frac{SD(e)^{a}}{SD(x)}$	R^{b}	Correction factor[c]	Estimate of β	Relative risk at 200 $\mu g/m^3$ years
0.00	1.00	1.00	0.018	4.6
0.10	0.99	1.02	0.018	4.7
0.20	0.96	1.04	0.019	4.9
0.30	0.92	1.09	0.021	5.3
0.40	0.86	1.16	0.024	5.9
0.50	0.80	1.25	0.029	6.8
0.75	0.64	3.27	0.059	12.8
1.00	0.50	20.00[d]	0.360[d]	73.0[d]
1.50	0.31	–	–	–
2.00	0.20	–	–	–

[a] Ratio of standard deviation of errors e to standard deviation of true exposures x.
[b] Reliability R of z as a measurement of x.
[c] See Eq. (9) in text.
[d] Model unrealistic, estimates unreliable for error of this magnitude and greater.

(see below). The results in Table 2, in particular those for higher SD(e), should thus be interpreted with caution.

Parallels with Misclassification

The general results given above are consistent with the well-known results for categorical (in particular dichotomous) exposure measures subject to misclassification that is "nondifferential" (equally likely in cases and noncases). Odds ratios are biased towards 1; tests for association remain valid but with reduced power compared with those using data without misclassification. See Kelsey et al. (1986) and Chen (1989) for reviews from an epidemiological and statistical perspective respectively.

A numerical exposure is often used to divide study subjects into several categories (bins), so that simple methods of estimating relative risks can be used. Accounting for errors may then be approached using either the misclassification or measurement error framework. The measurement error framework is probably more useful if the objective is to estimate the relationship between number of units of exposure and risk, in which case essentially the same results apply as for continuous numerical exposures (see also below).

Logistic and Other Binary Regression Models

Logistic and related models are often used for binary responses, for example in simple cohort studies with time to disease occurrence not observed. The effects of measurement error in these models are generally similar, but not identical, to those described above. More precise but considerably more computationally arduous methods of accounting for measurement error bias in these models are discussed by Carroll et al. (1984), Stefanski and Carroll (1985), Armstrong (1985), Schafer (1987), Whittemore and Grosser (1986), and others. When "logistic" regression is used to analyse case-control data, it is generally the (exponential) relative risk model which is assumed in the underlying population (Prentice and Farewell 1986), so that the simpler results for this model remain applicable, if the assumptions discussed above hold.

Other Measurement Error Models Arising in Occupational Cancer Epidemiology

Unfortunately, the simple models for measurement error described above rarely apply exactly to the data typically arising in occupational cancer epidemiology. Often the results from these simple models will be sufficiently valid to examine the possible impact of measurement error or otherwise aid interpretation even when assumptions are not met exactly, but if precise corrections are required, or if departures from model assumptions are substantial, other models should be considered. We discuss below some important situations in which this is so.

The Distribution of Measurement Error and of Exposures

The results above depend on measurement error and true exposures being distributed normally. This is clearly an imperfect model, since exposures are usually measured on a scale with an origin at zero. Further, the distributions of cumulative exposures to airborne contaminants and many other exposure measures thought to be relevant for occupational carcinogens are generally skewed to the right, often approximating to the lognormal distribution. Also measurement errors may be better represented in a multiplicative rather than additive model:

$$z = xe, \qquad \mathrm{E}(e) = 1 \tag{12}$$

One such model has measurement error following a lognormal distribution, so that:

$$\log(z) = \log(x) + \log(e) \tag{13}$$

Under this model, while taking logarithms has the effect of returning to the additive, normal distribution measurement and exposure model (and thus allowing the simple methods given above to be applied) exposures measured on the log scale will not be related to risk according to the same model that relates (original true) exposures to risk. Even if the model with logged exposures is as plausible as that with exposures on the original scale, the more difficult interpretation of parameters in the former will usually lead researchers to prefer the latter. Thus, in the preferred model exposures and measurement errors are lognormal, but relative risk is related to exposure on its original scale.

Estimating the true regression parameter in this model is more complex. The general approach of Prentice (1982) and Clayton (1988) leads to an estimator discussed by Armstrong and Oakes (1982), but the properties of this estimator remain to be explored. Although the naive test of $\beta_1^*=0$ using the crude data remains a valid test of $\beta_1=0$, it is no longer as powerful as some alternatives (Tosteson and Tsiatis 1988).

Nonnormal measurement error models may importantly alter the shape as well as the magnitude or the slope of relationships of relative risk to exposure (Prentice 1982). For example, Doll and Peto (1978) speculated that a quadratic relationship of lung cancer risk with true pack-years of exposure to tobacco smoke may be distorted to a linear form due to this type of measurement error.

Predictive and Structural Relationships

We have assumed in the above discussion that the parameter of interest is β_1, the "true" regression slope in the population, rather than β_1^*, the "naive" regression slope in the population. However, if the object of a study is to predict say relative risks in persons drawn from a population with the same distributions of true exposures and measurement error as the study group, then the naive β_1^* is the appropriate parameter, and standard uncorrected estimate of it may be made from the crude data. For this reason the regression involving β_1^* is called the "predictive" relationship in contrast to that involving β_1 which is known as the "structural", or in a slightly different context the "functional" relationship (Kendall and Stuart 1979).

When in occupational epidemiology we wish to predict risk we rarely wish to do so only for persons drawn from the same population with exposure measured with similar precision as the study group. In some situations (generally for discussions on setting standards) the structural relationship is clearly the one of interest. In others (e.g. predicting risk in workers from different populations) a predictive relationship is of interest, but not the same one as that estimated from the study. In the latter case the desired predictive relationship can be derived from the structural relationship using an inverse "correction for attenuation" appropriate for the new distributions of measurement error and true exposures. The original predictive relationship does seem the appropriate one for assessing compensability of cases, if risk (and hence probability of causation) is to be predicted for cases from the study group and exposure is measured using the same methods as for the study.

Classical and Berkson Models

The model, Eq. (2), in which error e is independent of x is generally called the classical measurement error model. An alternative (the Berkson model, after Berkson 1950) assumes that the error e is independent of the observed z. This is appropriate, for example, in experimental situations where the experimental sets the value of a variable to a nominal value (z), but the true value (x) may be in error in either direction (thus the model is sometimes called the "control-knob" model). Remarkably, in the exponential and linear relative risk regression models with normal measurement error of the Berkson type, the naive estimate $\hat{\beta}_1^*$ is unbiased for the true β_1, although random error is reflected in a higher standard error, and reduced power to test $\beta_1 = 0$ (Prentice 1982). Berkson type error does attenuate the regression parameter in a logistic model, but this bias is usually small compared with that due to classical measurement error. See Schafer et al. (1989) for results in the similar probit model.

It would seem at first that for occupational epidemiological studies that are not experimental the classical measurement error model is more appropriate than the Berkson model. However, this is not always the case. If for example a single estimate of concentration of exposure is taken to apply to all persons with the same job title, that error which is due to variation of individual workers exposures about this value is of the Berkson type. However, the single estimate of concentration of exposure is itself usually an approximation to the true mean concentration of exposures among men with the job title. The difference between this true mean and the exposure estimate constitutes "classical" measurement error. Thus, the many occupational epidemiological studies using this type of exposure estimation are generally subject to both Berkson and classical types of measurement error, only the latter causing attenuation in linear regression slopes. By a similar argument, the approximation involved in putting numerical continuous exposures into categories, and representing these categories in a regression by the mean exposures in each, introduces additional error of the Berkson type, but leaves the classical error structure essentially the same.

Differential Measurement Error

All the models discussed so far require the assumption that measurement error e is independent of disease status. For case-control studies in particular, recall or other information bias may act to create such a dependence. The qualitative effects of such error may be derived on common-sense grounds. Their effects and correction for them have been discussed formally for exposures which are normally distributed in cases and controls—the discriminant analysis model (Armstrong et al. 1989). Significance tests based on the crude data are not in this case valid tests of no association between true exposures and disease.

Cohort Studies Using Person Years at Risk Analyses and Standardized Mortality Ratios

The person-years at risk method of analysing cohort studies may be placed within the relative risk regression framework. Estimates of exposure-response relationships from internal person-years at risk analyses which assign numerical exposures to categories can thus be corrected for measurement error using the methods discussed above. However, the use of an external standard to calculate standardized mortality ratios (SMRs) gives additional information which can be useful in identifying and correcting measurement error effects.

Table 3 shows SMRs by cumulative exposure in miners exposed to tremolite fibers (McDonald et al. 1986). To estimate increment in risk per fiber-year (fy) we may fit a linear relationship to the observed SMRs and exposures (Hanley and Liddell 1985), giving $SMR = 1.52 + 0.011\,fy$. Expressed as a risk relative to that at zero exposure by dividing through by 1.52, we get $RR = 1 + 0.007\,fy$. If the reference rates are appropriate, so that an underlying SMR of 1.00 at zero exposure can be assumed, we may alternatively constrain the relationship to go through an SMR of 1.00 at zero exposure, giving $SMR\ (= RR) = 1.00 + 0.013\,fy$. This last approach is in any case more precise under this assumption, but it has added credibility and merit if measurement error is operating. Measurement error could explain the higher SMRs for lower exposure groups (which would in fact include some misclassified highly exposed persons) and the steeper constrained estimate of regression slope is consistent with attenuation of the unconstrained estimate due to measurement error. Putting aside some minor technical details and using Eq. (11) it can be shown that in this situation of relatively high mean risk in the study population, an attenuation of this magnitude would under a normal measurement error model follow from

Table 3. Standardized mortality ratios (SMRs) for respiratory cancer in miners exposed to mineral fibers[a]

Cumulative exposure (fy)	Mean cum. exp. in group[b]	Observed deaths	SMR (95% CI)
0–24	6	4	1.68(0.46–4.30)
25–199	77	3	1.85(0.38–5.41)
200–499	332	5	9.80(3.18–22,87)
500 +	836	3	6.77(1.40–19.79)
All	145	15	2.85(1.60–4.70)

[a] Including only years at risk at least 20 years from first employment (see McDonald et al. 1986).

[b] Mean among men terminating in this group, cumulated to end of service.

measurement reliability for cumulative exposure of about 0.75. The constrained estimate of exposure-response discussed above is very similar to a crude constrained estimate obtained by drawing a line between an SMR of 1.00 at 0 *fy* and that of 2.85 for the entire group (mean exp 145 *fy*). This may be shown to be an unbiased "instrumental variable" estimate; it also gives the relationship SMR (=RR)=1.00+0.013 *fy*. Both these constrained approaches trade measurement error bias off against the possibility of bias due to using an inappropriate reference.

Estimating the Measurement Error Distribution

Application of the simple corrections for attenuation of the regression parameter given above depend on the reliability R being known. Usually R itself must be estimated, ideally from a validity study in which approximate measures of exposure are compared with a "gold standard", or from a reliability study of repeated independent approximate measures of exposure in the same individuals. The way in which this should be done, and the manner in which uncertainties in the resulting estimate of R can be reflected in the estimate and more importantly the confidence intervals (and test results) of the regression parameter β_1 is the subject of much of the measurement error literature (Fuller 1987). We only have space to touch on some of the issues involved here.

Estimating R from a validation or reliability data set which is not a random sample from the main study population requires the assumption that not only the variance of measurement error, var (e), but also that of the true exposures, var(x), is the same as those in the main study. To avoid the latter assumption, we may estimate measurement error variance from the validation or reliability data set, and then use that estimate to estimate variance of true exposures and hence R from the distribution of approximate exposures observed in the main study. Where information from which R is estimated is not so substantial that uncertainties in R may be ignored, the simple methods given above should be refined so that this uncertainty can be reflected in wider confidence limits for the corrected estimate of β_1, for example by using the delta method to estimate var$(R\beta_1^*)$.

In occupational cancer epidemiology exposures must generally be estimated using retrospective hygiene surveys depending as much on hygienists' judgement as on any actual measures of available concentration of exposure available. "Gold standards" are almost never available. Estimates of exposure may be repeated, for example by different hygienists, and considered as a reliability study. However, it is difficult to envisage a situation in which such repeated estimates could be considered independent. The historical base of quantitative and qualitative information on which estimates must be based would be the same in each case; furthermore, a "random sample" of independent hygienists would be inconvenient to assemble, perhaps not even possible to conceive of. However, despite limitations, such studies can give important information on the possible magnitude of errors. At least one has been carried out for exposures retrospectively estimated in categories (Goldberg et al. 1986). Similar exercises do not seem to have been reported for quantitative retrospective exposure estimates.

Where more formal estimates of measurement error variance are unavailable, the best approach may be to carry out sensitivity analyses in which the consequences of measurement errors of various magnitudes are investigated, using the method in which R is assumed known. Choices of R used in these analyses may be informed by any data available, as well as general plausibility arguments. An alternative is to estimate the true regression parameter, using "instrumental" variables, a method which does not require any direct information on measurement error variance. However, although this has been discussed in some detail for regression models with numerical outcome variables (Kendall and Stuart 1979), its use for relative risk models remains largely unexplored.

Models with Many Explanatory Variables: Errors in Confounding Variables

Even when we are mainly interested in a single occupational risk factor, we often wish to control in the analysis for confounding by one or more nonoccupational factors – for example smoking habit. Furthermore, we may be interested in investigating several occupational exposures simultaneously. Much of the popularity of relative risk regression models lies in their capacity to carry out these functions, and to enable the investigation of interactions (effect modification).

Measurement error may be present in the observed occupational or nonoccupational factors. Although many of the statistical models for measurement error discussed above can be extended simply in theory to many variables, the computations required are generally substantially more involved, and most importantly the qualitative effects of measurement error on a specific variable can be quite different to those in the univariate case. Armstrong et al. (1989) discuss the exponential relative risk model with normal measurement error. The qualitative effect of measurement error in this model in one or both of two explanatory variables, which we shall interpret as being an occupational exposure of interest and a confounder, are discussed briefly below.

If the occupational exposure is subject to error, the regression parameter for this exposure is attenuated in a similar way to the univariate case, but this attenuation will be more accentuated. This accentuation of the attenuation (increase in bias) may be important, and occurs even if the nonoccupational factor is not actually associated with the disease (i.e. has been unnecessarily included as a confounder). This may occur in occupational studies when length of service is unnecessarily included as a possible confounder (to guard against "survivor effect" confounding) and interest is in a measure, for example cumulative exposure, which is strongly correlated with length of service. Of course, if length of service is a risk factor independently from the effect of cumulative exposure, not including it will introduce confounding bias, so that in the absence of methods for controlling measurement error bias the investigator must choose between the possibility of confounding bias and that of accentuated measurement error bias.

If the confounder is measured with error, then its inclusion in the regression can only partially control for its confounding effect. The "residual confounding" remaining may act to bias the regression parameter for the exposure of interest either way. If the exposure of interest is also subject to error, then this residual confounding is coupled with the accentuated attenuation discussed above. If the two errors are correlated, the extent and direction of the bias may be altered.

The effects of misclassification in dichotomous measures of an exposure of interest and a confounder have been discussed by Greenland (1980), and those of measurement error on partial correlation coefficients by Kupper (1984). These authors obtain similar qualitative results to those above. Greenland also observes that spurious interactions between variables may be introduced by misclassification, a result which seems likely to apply also to numerical measures of exposure subject to random error.

Discussion

This brief overview could not include reference to many important advances in methods available to address the effects to measurement error on estimates of exposure-response relationships. However, for the structures of measurement error common in occupational cancer epidemiology, there remains much work to be done before fully appropriate methods are sufficiently established for ready application by epidemiologists. In the meantime, ad hoc arguments concerning the likely impact of measurement error may usefully be based on the results from simpler models described above and elsewhere.

References

Armstrong BG (1985) Measurement error in the generalised linear model. Comm Statist Simul Comp 14: 529–544

Armstrong BG, Oakes D (1982) The effects of approximation in exposure assessments on estimates of exposure response relationships. Scand J Work Environ Health 8 [Suppl 1]: 20–23

Armstrong BG, Tremblay CG, Cyr D, Thériault GP (1986) Estimating the relationship between exposure to tar volatiles and the incidence of bladder cancer in aluminum smelter workers. Scand J Work Environ Health 12: 486–493

Armstrong BG, Whittemore AS, Howe GR (1989) Analysis of case-control data with covariate measurement error: application to diet and colon cancer. Stat Med 8: 1151–1165

Berkson J (1950) Are there two regressions? J Am Stat Assoc 45: 164–180

Carroll RJ, Spiegelman CH, Lan KK, Bailey KT, Abbott RD (1984) On errors-in-variables for binary regression models. Biometrika 71: 19–25

Chen TT (1989) Overview of misclassification in epidemiology. Stat Med 8: 1095–1106
Clayton DG (1988) Models for the analysis of cohort and case-control studies with inaccurately measured exposures. In: Dwyer JH, Lippert P, Feinleib M, Hoffmeister H (eds) Statistical models for longitudinal studies of health. Oxford University Press, New York
Cochran WG (1968) Errors of measurement in statistics. Technometrics 10: 637–666
Doll R, Peto R (1978) Cigarette smoking and bronchial carcinoma: dose and time relationships among regular and lifelong nonsmokers. J Epidemiol Community Health 32: 303–313
Fuller WA (1987) Measurement error models. Wiley, New York
Goldberg MS, Siemiatycki J, Gerin M (1986) Inter-rater agreement in assessing occupational exposure in a case-control study. Br J Ind Med 43: 667–676
Greenland S (1980) The effect of misclassification in the presence of covariates. Am J Epidemiol 112: 564–569
Hanley J, Liddell FDK (1985) Fitting relationships between exposure and standardized mortality ratios. J Occup Med 27: 555–560
Kelsey JL, Thompson WD, Evans AS (1986) Methods in observational epidemiology. Oxford University Press, New York, pp 285–308
Kendall M, Stuart A (1979) The advanced theory of statistics vol 2. MacMillan, New York, pp 399–443
Kupper L (1984) Effects of the use of unreliable surrogate variables on the validity of epidemiological research studies. Am J Epidemiol 120: 643–648
Lagakos S (1987) Effects of mismodelling and mismeasuring explanatory variables on tests of their association with a response variable. Stat Med 7: 257–274
McDonald JC, McDonald AD, Armstrong BG, Sebastien P (1986) Cohort mortality study of vermiculite miners exposed to tremolite. Br J Ind Med 43: 436–444
Pepe M, Self SG, Prentice RL (1989) Further results on covariate measurement errors in cohort studies with time to response data. Stat Med 8: 1167–1178
Prentice RL (1982) Covariate measurement error and parameter estimation in a failure time regression model. Biometrika 69: 331–342
Prentice RL, Farewell VT (1986) Relative risk and odds ratio regression. Annu Rev Public Health 7: 35–58
Schafer DW (1987) Covariate measurement error in generalised linear models. Biometrika 74: 385–391
Schafer DW, Stefanski LA, Tosteson TD (1989) A measurement error model for binary and ordinal regression. Stat Med 8: 1139–1138
Snedecor GW, Cochran WG (1967) Statistical methods. Iowa State University Press, Iowa, pp 164–167
Stefanski LA, Carroll RJ (1985) Covariate measurement error in logistic regression. Ann Stat 13: 1335–1351
Thériault G, Tremblay C, Cordier S, Gingras S (1984) Bladder cancer in the aluminium industry. Lancet i: 947–950
Tosteson TD, Tsiatis AA (1988) The asymptotic relative efficiency of score tests in the generalized linear model with surrogate covariates. Biometrika 75: 507–514
Whittemore AS, Grosser S (1986) Regression methods for data with incomplete covariates. In: Moolgavkar SH, Prentice RR (eds) Modern statistical methods in chronic disease epidemiology. Wiley, New York, pp 19–34
Willett W (1989) An epidemiologic perspective on exposure measurement error. Stat Med 8: 1031–1040

Adjustment for Confounding in Occupational Cancer Epidemiology

J.J. Spinelli, P.R. Band, and R.P. Gallagher

Division of Epidemiology, Biometry and Occupational Oncology, Cancer Control Agency of British Columbia, 600 West 10th Avenue, Vancouver, B.C. V5Z 4E6, Canada

The historical cohort mortality study, the most common method for determining occupational cancer risk factors, is usually conducted without adjusting for important confounding variables, such as smoking. This is because obtaining data on confounders is often costly and difficult. To what extent this lack of information is likely to cause serious bias in the estimation of occupation-disease relationships is the object of this paper.

Confounding is a bias that occurs in the estimation of the effect of an exposure on disease occurrence; due to the association of another factor with both the disease and the exposure. A confounder, then, is any factor that when properly controlled, gives an estimate of a causal parameter that is closer to the true value. To be a confounder a factor must meet two criteria, it must be a risk factor for the disease in the unexposed population, and it must be associated with the exposure of interest.

The degree of confounding can be expressed quantitatively as follows. Let I_c and $I_{\bar{c}}$ be the incidence rates of a disease in the presence and the absence of a particular potential confounding factor. And let I_e and $I_{\bar{e}}$ be the incidence rates of a disease in the presence and absence of an exposure. Let R_c be the incidence rate ratio (or risk ratio) due to the factor, which is the ratio of the incidence rate in the presence of the factor to the incidence rate in the absence of the factor ($I_c/I_{\bar{c}}$). Also, let R_e be the true risk ratio for the exposure, and P_{ce} and $P_{c\bar{e}}$ be the proportion with the factor in the exposed and unexposed populations. Then, the risk ratio for the exposure unadjusted for the effect of the factor which I will refer to as R_{eu}, (u standing for unadjusted), is

$$\begin{aligned} R_{eu} &= I_e/I_{\bar{e}} \\ &= R_e \frac{[I_c P_{ce} + I_{\bar{c}}\,(1-P_{ce})]}{I_c P_{c\bar{e}} + I_{\bar{c}}\,(1-P_{c\bar{e}})} \\ &= R_e \frac{[R_c I_{\bar{c}} P_{ce} + I_{\bar{c}}\,(1-P_{ce})]}{R_c I_{\bar{c}} P_{c\bar{e}} + I_{\bar{c}}\,(1-P_{c\bar{e}})]} \\ &= R_e \frac{[(R_c-1)P_{ce}+1]}{(R_c-1)P_{c\bar{e}}+1} \end{aligned} \tag{1}$$

Recent Results in Cancer Research, Vol. 120

The degree of confounding can be measured by the ratio of the unadjusted risk ratio, R_{eu}, and the true (or adjusted) risk ratio, R_e, and has been labelled the confounding risk ratio, or *CRR* by Miettinen (1972). Substituting the right-hand side of Eq. (1) for the unadjusted risk ratio gives

$$CRR = \frac{R_{eu}}{R_e} = \frac{(R_c - 1)P_{ce} + 1}{(R_c - 1)P_{c\bar{e}} + 1} \qquad (2)$$

R_{eu} substantially different from R_e, or equivalently, the confounding risk ratio much different from one, implies that the factor is a confounder for the exposure of interest.

Note that if the risk ratio due to the factor, R_c, equals one, or if the proportion with the factor in the exposed and unexposed populations is equal ($P_{ce} = P_{c\bar{e}}$) then the confounding risk ratio equals one, and the factor is not a confounder. This agrees with the definition that a confounder must be related to the disease and related to the exposure of interest. Also, the right-hand side of Eq. (2) provides a method of indirectly estimating the confounding effect of a factor without information on the exposure-disease association.

Two assumptions were made in the derivation of the confounding risk ratio. The first assumption is that the effect of the confounding factor and the exposure act multiplicatively on the risk of disease. That is, the risk ratio in the presence of both the confounder and the exposure is equal to the risk ratio for the confounder times the true risk ratio for the exposure. The definition of the confounding risk ratio under an additive risk model will not be considered in this article, but is discussed in a paper by Gail et al. (1988). The second assumption is that the true risk ratio for the exposure is not influenced by the level or value of the confounding factor. The violation of this assumption is referred to as interaction or effect modification. These assumptions can only be tested by direct estimation of the effect at each level of the exposure and confounding factor. Two other points need to be considered. First, by substituting the rates and proportions of the general population for those in the unexposed group, we obtain the risk ratios for a standard cohort study in which the incidence or mortality rate in the exposed group is compared with that of the general population. Second, the calculation of the confounding risk ratio can be easily extended to confounders with more than two levels by allowing different risks and prevalence rates for each level of the confounder. If in fact, the risk ratio varies among different levels of the confounding factor and these levels are not taken into account in estimating the true risk ratio, R_e, then the risk ratio will be biased. The degree of this bias depends on the variability in the risk ratio for the different levels of the confounder not being taken into account (Breslow and Day 1980).

It has been shown that the confounding risk ratio is considerably less than either the association of the confounder with the disease or the association of the confounder with the exposure (Breslow and Day 1980). Thus, only those factors with a strong association with the disease of interest and with large differential prevalence rates across particular occupations will be major confounders in occupational studies.

Clearly, the factor with the largest association to diseases of importance in occupational studies is smoking and the disease with the largest smoking association is lung cancer. Smoking is also causally related to several other diseases including nonmalignant lung diseases, other types of cancer, and coronary heart disease, which have also been related to occupation.

Axelson provided evidence of the degree of smoking confounding in occupational cancer studies by constructing Table 1 showing the potential confounding risk ratios for hypothetical populations compared with a referent group approximating the smoking rates for the Swedish population (Axelson 1978). To obtain a confounding risk ratio due to smoking of greater than 3, a population with 100% heavy smokers is needed. As well, a confounding risk ratio greater than 2 requires a population with no nonsmokers and 35% heavy smokers. Similarly, confounding risk ratios of less than 0.5 are only obtained for populations with no heavy smokers. In view of these results, observed occupational risk ratios of greater than 2 are unlikely to be due entirely to confounding by smoking. However, any occupation-disease association with a risk ratio less than 2 could be totally confounded by smoking.

Very large relative risks for lung cancer were attributed to moderate and heavy smokers. For smaller relative risks, the confounding risk ratios would be closer to one. Thus, other potential confounding factors with smaller relative risks, socioeconomic status, for example, or the effect of smoking on other causes of death, such as coronary heart disease or bladder cancer are likely to have confounding risk ratios much closer to one.

Table 1. Confounding risk ratios (CRR) for smoking in estimation of the risk ratio (RR) for lung cancer (from Axelson 1978)

Percentage of group			
Non-smoker (RR = 1)	Moderate smoker (RR = 10)	Heavy smoker (RR = 20)	CRR
100	0	0	0.15
80	20	0	0.43
60	35	5	0.78
50[a]	40	10	1.00
40	45	15	1.22
20	55	25	1.65
10	60	30	1.86
0	65	35	2.08
0	0	100	3.08

[a] Referent population.

It is apparent that for significant smoking confounding to exist, the occupational group studied needs to have a very different smoking profile than the general population. Several studies have been published examining the smoking habits of different occupational groups. Table 2 presents data from the 1985 report from the U.S. Surgeon General which showed that the percentage of current smokers among male workers ranged from 55% for painters, construction and maintenance workers to 16% for electrical workers and electrical engineers. Substituting these rates into the equation for the confounding risk ratio, using the general population smoking rate of 41%, and assigning a risk ratio for lung cancer for current smokers of ten, gives a range of confounding risk ratios of 0.53 to 1.27.

Additional information on the range of smoking in occupational groups comes from a study by Asp who surveyed the smoking habits of 1990 males participating in a health screening program in Finland, and found that the percentage of current smokers ranged from a high of 68%–74% in mobile machine operators and construction workers, to a low of 22%–30% in civil servants, and business executives (Table 3) (Asp 1984). This study offers the improvement of examining smoking in three categories: never, ex, and current smoker. Using Asp's study population as the comparison group, the confounding risk ratio for smoking varied from 0.67 for civil servants to 1.31 for construction workers.

The previous two studies were examples of indirect estimation of the confounding risk ratios. Studies have also been conducted which directly estimate the confounding risk ratio for smoking by examining unadjusted and smoking-adjusted risk ratios. This direct approach has the advantage that it does not require a prior assumption about the risk ratio for the confounder, but estimates it directly for the population of interest. However, the disadvantage is that the estimates of the crude and adjusted risk ratios are subject to sampling error.

Blair et al. (1985) directly estimated the confounding effect of smoking using data from a cohort study of 294000 white male U.S. veterans. They examined

Table 2. Confounding risk ratios (CRR) for smoking in estimation of the risk ratio (RR) for lung cancer (from US Surgeon General 1985)

	Percentage current smokers	CRR (RR = 10)
Electrical workers and electrical engineers	16.2	0.53
Population	40.9	1.00
Painters, construction and maintenance workers	55.1	1.27

Table 3. Confounding risk ratios (CRR) for smoking in estimation of the risk ratio (RR) for lung cancer. (From Asp 1984)

Occupational group	Non-smoker (RR=1)	Percentage exsmoker (RR=10)	Current smoker (RR=20)	CRR
Civil servants	41	37	22	0.67
Business executives	30	40	30	0.81
Total population	24	28	48	1.00
Mobile machine operators	7	25	68	1.28
Construction workers	10	16	74	1.31

Table 4. Confounding risk ratios (CRR) for smoking in estimation of the standardized mortality ratio (SMR) for lung cancer. (From Blair et al. 1985)

Occupational group	Crude SMR	Adjusted SMR	CRR
Tailors and upholsterers	0.93	1.44	0.65
Bakers and cooks	1.57	2.25	0.70
Editors and reporters	1.09	0.79	1.37
Tinsmiths and sheet-metal workers	1.36	0.94	1.45

smoking in four categories: never smokers, ex-smokers, current cigarette smokers and smokers of other tobacco products or with missing smoking information. Usual occupation was the exposure variable examined. In order to minimize the sampling variability, they excluded occupations with less than five observed and expected deaths.

Table 4 shows the crude and adjusted standardized mortality ratios (SMRs) and confounding risk ratios for the occupations with the most extreme confounding risk ratios. The smallest confounding risk ratios were found for tailors and upholsterers (0.65) and bakers and cooks (0.70). The largest confounding risk ratios were for tinsmiths and sheet-metal workers (1.45) and for editors and reporters (1.37). Notice that for editors and reporters and tinsmiths and sheet-metal workers the crude SMRs were greater than one and the adjusted SMRs were less than one. Also, the crude SMR was less than one and the adjusted SMR greater than one for tailors and upholsterers. In these situations, the unadjusted SMR estimate would incorrectly assess the occupation-lung cancer relationship.

In a recently published report, Siemiatycki et al. (1988) looked at crude and adjusted odds ratios for occupation and lung cancer from a study of 791 lung cancer cases and 2063 other cancer and population controls, providing additional information on smoking confounding by directly estimating the confounding bias of smoking in a case-control study. The report also assessed the effect of degree of smoking stratification on the estimation of the confounding bias by examining several smoking classifications with different degrees of stratification. Among the smoking variables examined were never smoker vs ever smoker, and cumulative amount of cigarettes smoked in three and five levels.

Exposure in this study was defined as working in a particular occupation for more than 6 months. To minimize the effect of sampling variation, only the 25 occupations with the most subjects were considered.

The measure of the confounding effect utilized was the confounding bias factor rather than the confounding risk ratio. The confounding bias factor is defined as the ratio of the unadjusted to the adjusted odds ratio, or the ratio of the adjusted to the unadjusted odds ratio, whichever is greater. This was done because the investigators felt that the extent of confounding was more important than the direction of the confounding. Because for certain smoking categories only the confounding bias factor was reported, the magnitude of negative and positive confounding cannot be evaluated. The level of the confounding bias factor for each of the 25 occupations studied by Siemiatycki and his colleagues is shown in Table 5. The largest confounding bias factor was 1.62, for teachers. No other occupation had a confounding bias factor greater than 1.30 and, for the five-level smoking adjustment, 21 of 25 or 84%, were less than 1.20.

The data suggest that the greater the degree of smoking stratification the greater the confounding bias factor. The proportion of occupations with a confounding bias factor greater than 1.20 are 1 of 25 or 4% for both the never/ever smoking variable and the three-level cumulative amount smoking variable and 4 of 25 or 16% for the five-level cumulative amount smoking variable. Additional information on smoking confounding in occupational

Table 5. Number of occupations with indicated confounding bias factors by smoking stratification in the estimation of the risk ratio for lung cancer. (From Siemiatycki et al. 1988)

Confounding bias factor	Never/ ever	Pack years (3 levels)	Pack years (5 levels)
1.00–1.10	20	13	10
1.11–1.20	4	11	11
1.21–1.30	1	0	3
1.31–1.40	0	0	0
1.41–1.50	0	0	0
1.51–1.62	0	1	1

cancer studies is provided from two studies conducted at the Cancer Control Agency of British Columbia; an historical cohort study of aluminum workers and a population based case-control study examining occupational risk factors.

The cohort study of aluminum workers includes all workers with 3 or more years experience at the Alcan aluminum plant in Kitimat, British Columbia. The mortality and cancer incidence of these workers will be compared with that of the British Columbia population. The primary contaminant of interest is polycyclic aromatic hydrocarbons or PAHs and the major suspected cancer risks from exposure to PAHs are lung and bladder cancer. We have identified 6210 individuals as past or current employees with 3 or more years of experience of whom 2127 are active employees. Data collected on each individual include identifying information and a complete work history. Smoking information is also being collected on each worker, and comes from four sources, self-reported (62%), next-of-kin (7%), collected information from a 1981 respiratory disease study conducted by the University of British Columbia (Chan-Yeung et al. 1983) (30%), and company health records (1%). Smoking information is still being collected, but complete smoking information (defined as known smoking status (non, ex, or current smoker) and usual amount of cigarettes smoked) is available for 75% of the total cohort and 86% of the active employees at this time. The follow-up of the cohort is not yet complete, but the potential confounding effect due to smoking in estimation of the lung cancer risk can be indirectly estimated using the available smoking information.

The smoking distributions for the British Columbia population, obtained from Health and Welfare Canada's 1983 Labour Force Survey (Jassa 1983), for the total cohort and for the active employees in the cohort are in Table 6. In British Columbia, never smokers comprise 43% of the population, ex-smokers 28% and current smokers 29% of which 6% are heavy smokers. The smoking rates of the cohort are higher than that of the general population, as there are fewer never smokers (26%), more ex-smokers (38%) and more moderate and heavy smokers, 21% and 8%. The formula for indirectly assessing the confounding risk ratio was applied using the following risk ratios for lung cancer mortality; 10 for ex and light smokers, 15 for moderate smokers and 25 for heavy smokers. This results in a confounding risk ratio of 1.26, which indicates that SMRs of 1.30 or greater for lung cancer cannot be explained by a differential smoking distribution. Direct estimates of the smoking-adjusted SMR and tests for interaction effects will be made upon completion of the study.

The smoking rates of the active cohort were examined to determine the effect of using a sample of active workers from whom information is easier to obtain in order to indirectly assess confounding. This is a useful technique if the smoking distribution of the active workers approximates the smoking distribution of the entire cohort. As shown in Table 6, active employees smoke slightly more than former employees with 24% and 10% moderate and heavy smokers respectively. Using this information, a confounding risk ratio of 1.32 was obtained. This estimate is similar although slightly higher to that obtained from

Table 6. Confounding risk ratio (CRR) for smoking in estimation of the risk ratio (RR) for lung cancer in the cohort of aluminum workers

	Never smoker	Percentage Ex-smoker	Current smoker (cig/day)			CRR
			< 10	11–25	26+	
RR=	1	10	10	15	25	
B.C. population (males 1983)	42.9	28.5	7.2	15.2	6.2	
Total cohort	26.2	37.6	7.1	21.0	8.0	1.26
Active cohort	26.6	31.3	7.9	23.8	10.2	1.32

the smoking data from the entire cohort, indicating that smoking information from current employees yields a reasonable indirect estimate of smoking confounding.

The remainder of the paper will focus on the results derived from a project referred to as the "Health in the Workplace Study," a population-based occupational case-control study. All male cancer cases in British Columbia aged 20 years and over have, since 1983, received a questionnaire requesting detailed information on work and smoking history. To this date over 14000 questionnaires have been collected. Substantive results from this study are presented elsewhere in this volume (Band et al.).

The data used for the analysis of smoking confounding were 715 squamous cell lung cancer cases collected over the first 4 years of the study, and 1430 other cancer controls, matched 2:1 on 5-year age group and year of identification. The objectives to this analysis were first to provide independent evidence of the extent of smoking confounding in occupational cancer studies, and second to determine the confounding effect of different levels of smoking stratification. Exposure was defined as more than 1 year employment in a particular occupation or industry. Occupations and industries were coded according to the 1981 Canadian Standard Occupational Classification and Standard Industrial Classification, respectively (Statistics Canada 1981a,b). Three-digit occupational and two-digit industrial groups were examined, for a total of 55 occupations and 76 industries.

In order to reduce the effect of sampling variation on confounding bias, only occupations and industries with at least 5 cancer cases or 10 controls were included in the analysis, for a total of 52 occupations and 60 industries. A greater restriction would have further reduced sampling variation, but might have eliminated jobs with extreme smoking distributions.

The effect of confounding was examined according to three different levels of smoking stratification. The first used three categories: never smoker, ever cigarette smoker and smokers of other tobacco products and unknown smoking status. The second consisted of four categories, with ever cigarette smokers separated into 1–30 and over 30 pack years. For the final stratification, ever cigarette smokers were separated into three categories, 1–24, 25–49 and 50 or more pack years. Table 7 presents the smoking distribution of the control group.

The proportion of never smokers in the control group was 18%, much lower than the 43% of the B.C. population which had never smoked as seen in Table 6. This is likely due to the inclusion of smoking related cancer sites, such as oral cavity and esophagus, in the control group. Four percent smoked other tobacco products only and 0.3% had unknown smoking status. In the four-level smoking classification, the percentages in the low and high cumulative amount of cigarettes smoked were 33% and 37% respectively, and for the five-level grouping 26%, 25% and 20% fell in the low, moderate and high categories respectively. Of the controls 8% had missing information on duration or intensity of cigarette smoking and were grouped with the unknown and other smokers for the analysis of the four- and five-level smoking classifications. Unadjusted and adjusted odds ratios used in the calculation of confounding risk ratios were estimated by conditional logistic regression using the program PECAN on a Sun 3 minicomputer running UNIX (Storer et al. 1983).

Table 8 shows the number of occupations with various confounding risk ratios by level of smoking stratification. The confounding risk ratios for the five-level smoking classification ranged from 0.47 to 1.50. Of the 52 occupations 11 or 21% had a confounding risk ratio outside of the middle range 0.80–1.25, and only two occupations had confounding risk ratios outside the range of 0.67–1.5. The dispersion of the confounding risk ratio increased slightly with the degree of smoking stratification, the standard deviations being 0.13, 0.17, and 0.19, respectively, for the three smoking groupings. Also, the proportion of occupations with confounding risk ratios outside the middle range 0.80–1.25,

Table 7. Percentage of controls in smoking categories from the Health in the Workplace Study

	3[a]		4		5	
Never smoker		18.0		18.0		18.0
Pack years (cigarette)	All	78.0	1–30	32.9	1–24	26.2
			31+	37.3	25–49	24.6
					50+	19.5
Other smoker (pipe, cigar)		3.7		3.7		3.7
Unknown smoking status		0.3		8.0		8.0

[a] Number of levels of smoking stratification.

Table 8. Number of occupations with indicated confounding risk ratios (CRR) by smoking stratification

	Levels of smoking stratification		
CRR	3	4	5
0.46–0.56	1	1	1
0.57–0.66	0	0	1
0.67–0.79	2	3	4
0.80–0.90	5	5	4
0.91–0.99	9	13	14
1.00	4	4	1
1.01–1.10	23	13	13
1.11–1.25	8	11	9
1.26–1.50	0	1	5
1.51–1.75	0	1	0
Mean	1.01	1.01	1.02
S.D.	0.13	0.17	0.19

Table 9. Odds ratios for selected occupations and lung cancer, unadjusted and adjusted for smoking

Occupation	SOC[a]	n[b]	$_{u}OR$[c]	$_{a}OR_3$[d]	$_{a}OR_4$[d]	$_{a}OR_5$[d]	CRR[e]
Apparel service	616	7	2.33	4.85	5.05	4.89	0.47
Processing[f]	815–816	19	1.73	1.94	2.12	2.69	0.64
Forestry	751	79	1.08	1.07	0.93	0.87	1.24
Water transport	915	38	1.29	1.09	0.98	1.00	1.29
Health professionals	311	3	0.27	0.26	0.24	0.18	1.50

[a] Canadian Standard Occupational Classification.
[b] Number of lung cancer cases who worked more than 1 year in the specific occupation.
[c] Unadjusted odds ratio.
[d] Odds ratio adjusted for the 3, 4, and 5 level smoking classifications, respectively.
[e] Ratio of the unadjusted odds ratio to the five-level smoking adjusted odds ratio ($_{u}OR/_{a}OR_5$).
[f] Chemicals/petroleum/rubber/plastics.

increased with increasing smoking stratification, as there were 3 of 52 or 6% for the three-level grouping, 6 or 12% for the four-level stratification and 11 or 21%, for the five-level classification.

The unadjusted and adjusted odds ratios for occupations with extreme confounding risk ratios are shown in Table 9. The smallest confounding risk ratios, 0.47 and 0.64, were observed for apparel service occupations, for example, dry cleaners, and for processing occupations in chemicals, petroleum, rubber or plastics. Most of the confounding in the apparel service occupations was accounted for by the three-level smoking classification, as the adjusted odds ratio was twice as large as the unadjusted one. Further smoking adjustment had little effect. However, the opposite was found for the processing occupations as the odds ratios increased steadily with increasing smoking stratification. Forestry and water transport occupations both had unadjusted odds ratios greater than 1.0 which steadily decreased to 1.0 or lower after adjustment for smoking. Health professionals had the largest confounding risk ratio, as the small unadjusted odds ratio became even smaller with increasing smoking stratification.

The results for industries revealed similar patterns. The confounding risk ratios for the five-level smoking stratification ranged from 0.63 to 1.68. Out of the 60 industries, 14 or 23% had confounding risk ratios outside the middle range 0.80–1.25 (compared with 21% for the occupations), and four had confounding risk ratios outside the range of 0.67–1.5 (compared with two for the occupations), shown in Table 10. The dispersion of the confounding risk ratio again increased with greater smoking stratification. The percentage of industries with confounding risk ratios outside the middle range were 4 of 60 or 7% for the three-level smoking stratification, 10 or 17% for the four-level grouping and 14 or 23% for the five-level classification. The standard deviations for the three levels of smoking stratification were 0.12, 0.19 and 0.21, respectively.

The unadjusted and adjusted odds ratios for the industries with the most extreme confounding risk ratios are shown in Table 11. The personal service industry which includes barbers and dry cleaners and the mineral products industry, for example, concrete products, had the smallest confounding risk

Table 10. Number of industries with indicated confounding risk ratios by smoking stratification

	Levels of smoking stratification		
CRR	3	4	5
0.57–0.66	1	3	1
0.67–0.79	3	3	7
0.80–0.90	7	12	9
0.91–0.99	17	11	8
1.00	2	1	6
1.01–1.10	23	19	12
1.11–1.25	7	7	11
1.26–1.50	0	2	3
1.51–1.75	0	2	3
Mean	1.00	1.00	1.02
S.D.	0.12	0.19	0.21

Table 11. Odds ratios for selected industries and lung cancer, unadjusted and adjusted for smoking

Industry	SIC	n	$_{u}OR$	$_{a}OR_3$	$_{a}OR_4$	$_{a}OR_5$	CRR
Personal Service	97	22	1.63	2.27	2.53	2.55	0.63
Mineral Products	35	7	0.93	1.06	1.05	1.30	0.71
Food Service	92	33	2.15	2.02	1.83	1.62	1.32
Storage	47	6	1.33	1.10	0.91	0.87	1.52
Banking	70	19	1.23	1.11	0.81	0.73	1.68

SIC, Canadian Standard Industrial Classification; for definition of other column headings, see Table 9.

ratios, 0.63 and 0.71 respectively. The five-level smoking-adjusted odds ratio for mineral products was 1.3, whereas the three- and four-level smoking adjusted odds ratios were close to one and the unadjusted odds ratio was less than one, 0.93, showing a change from an estimated reduced risk to an estimated increased risk. This represents an example of an increased risk which would have been missed in a cohort study without a finely stratified smoking adjustment. The odds ratios for the food service industry, that is, restaurants and taverns, steadily declined with increasing smoking stratification, giving a confounding risk ratio of 1.32, but the odds ratio after the five-level smoking adjustment remained elevated at 1.62. This exemplifies the situation where a large smoking confounding effect does not totally explain the unadjusted excess risk. The storage industry, which includes grain elevators, and the banking industry had the largest confounding risk ratios with moderate unadjusted odds ratios of 1.33 and 1.23 steadily dropping to less than one after adjusting for increasing smoking stratification. An odds ratio which changed from greater than one to less than one after adjustment was uncommon, as it occurred for only three occupations and four industries. However, it is important as it illustrates the situation where an excess risk would be erroneously reported if no smoking adjustment was made.

Table 12 summarizes the results of the studies discussed which examined the confounding effect of smoking in estimation of the occupation-lung cancer relationship in a range of occupations or industries. There are two conclusions to be drawn from this table. The first is that the studies show consistency in the range of confounding risk ratios with all falling being between 0.46 and 1.68. This indicates first that an odds ratio greater than 1.70, would be very unlikely to be confounded by cigarette smoking, and second that for an observed unadjusted odds ratio of one, the true odds ratio would not likely be greater than 2.2, a situation which would arise with a confounding risk ratio of 0.46.

The final conclusion is that the range of the confounding risk ratio, and particularly the highest value, increases with the degree of smoking stratification. Confounding risk ratios calculated from smoking variables of two or three

Table 12. Range of confounding risk ratios (CRR) for smoking in estimation of the relative risk for lung cancer

Study	Levels of smoking stratification	CRR range
U.S. Surgeon General (1985)	2	0.53–1.27
Asp (1984)	3	0.67–1.31
Blair et al. (1985)	4	0.67–1.45
Siemiatycki et al. (1988)	2	(0.77–1.30)
	3	0.62–1.19
	5	(0.62–1.62)
Health in the Workplace (occupation)	3	0.48–1.22
	4	0.46–1.61
	5	0.47–1.50
Health in the Workplace (industry)	3	0.61–1.25
	4	0.61–1.53
	5	0.63–1.68

levels such as in the reports of the U.S. Surgeon General, Siemiatycki et al., or our Health in the Workplace study show confounding risk ratios of less than 1.30. Analyses using a higher degree of smoking stratification show larger confounding risk ratios, as is particularly evident by our own results. This demonstrates that adjusting for smoking by a dichotomous variable could lead to biased estimates of the risk ratio, as not all confounding would be accounted for.

References

Asp S (1984) Confounding by variable smoking habits in different occupational groups. Scand J Work Environ Health 10: 325–326

Axelson O (1978) Aspects on confounding in occupational health epidemiology. Scand J Work Environ Health 4: 85–89

Blair A, Hoar S, Walrath J (1985) Comparison of crude and smoking-adjusted standardized mortality ratios. J Occup Med 27: 881–884

Breslow NE, Day NE (1980) Statistical methods in cancer research, vol 1. The analysis of case-control studies. International Agency for Research on Cancer, Lyon (IARC sci publ no 32)

Chan-Yeung M, Wong R, MacLean L, Tan F, Schulzer M, Enarson D, Martin A, Dennis R, Grzybowski S (1983) Epidemiologic health study of workers in an alumi-

num smelter in British Columbia: effects on the respiratory system. Am Rev Respir Dis 127: 465–469
Gail MH, Wacholder S, Lubin JH (1988) Indirect corrections for confounding under multiplicative and additive risk models. Am J Ind Med 13: 119–130
Jassa D (1983) Smoking behaviour of Canadians. Supply and Services Canada, Ottawa
Miettinen OS (1972) Components of the crude risk ratio. Am J Epidemiol 96: 168–172
Siemiatycki J, Wacholder S, Dewar R, Cardis E, Greenwood C, Richardson L (1988) Degree of confounding bias related to smoking, ethnic group and socioeconomic status in estimates of the associations between occupation and cancer. J Occup Med 30: 617–625
Statistics Canada (1981a) Standard occupational classification 1980. Statistics Canada, Ottawa (catalogue 12–565; ISBN 0–660–10672–8)
Statistics Canada (1981b) Standard industrial classification 1980. Statistics Canada, Ottawa (catalogue 12–501; ISBN 0–660–10672–8)
Storer BE, Wacholder S, Breslow NE (1983) Maximum likelihood fitting of general risk models to stratified data. Appl Stat 32: 177–181
US Surgeon General (1985) The health consequences of smoking, cancer and chronic lung disease in the workplace. Department of Health and Human Services, Rockville Md.

*Statistical Issues in the Analysis of Data from Occupational Cohort Studies**

N. Breslow

Department of Biostatistics, SC-32, University of Washington, Seattle, WA 98195, USA

The overwhelming majority of statistical analyses of occupational cohort data are conducted in terms of the standardized mortality ratio or SMR. Saracci and Johnson (1987) reviewed 55 cancer epidemiology papers published during 1982 in the *American Journal of Epidemiology*, the *British Journal of Industrial Medicine* and the *Journal of Occupational Medicine*. All but one of 20 occupational cohort studies that they identified employed the SMR as the principal method of analysis. In spite of its evident popularity, the SMR is particularly susceptible to the selection and confounding biases that affect observational studies generally (Hill 1953; Cochran 1983) and its uncritical use as a summary measure has received frequent criticism (e.g., Gaffey 1976). The continuing debate regarding the relative advantages of local vs national rates as a basis for comparison (Gardner 1986) is a reminder that many other factors besides membership in a particular occupational cohort affect disease rates. "Background" variation in SMRs computed for cohorts in different geographic areas can be expected to swamp the Poisson sampling variability that is reflected in the usual measures of statistical uncertainty.

Doubts about the validity of SMR analyses and the desire to make fuller use of the available data have stimulated the recent development of several alternative methods of analysis of occupational cohort data. Greater emphasis is now given to within cohort comparisons of disease rates, to control of confounding through multiple regression analysis and to mathematical modelling of dose-time-response relationships (Thomas 1988). These methods are reviewed in a recent monograph on the design and analysis of cohort studies (Breslow and Day 1987), from which much of the material in this paper is drawn.

Factors Affecting Disease Risk

Appropriate statistical analysis of data from any observational study requires careful consideration of factors that could influence the outcome measure so

* Paper prepared for the International Symposium on Occupational Cancer Epidemiology, Vancouver B.C., 13–13 June 1988. Supported in part by USPHS grant CA40644.

Recent Results in Cancer Research, Vol. 120

that their effects may be controlled to the greatest possible extent. Other factors may *modify* the primary associations of interest in such a way as to influence the causal interpretation. Relevant factors for occupational cohort studies include the following.

Age and Calendar Year at Follow-Up

These are the only factors controlled for in a standard SMR analysis. Age serves as a surrogate for cumulative nonspecific exposures, as well as changes in host susceptibility due to the aging process per se, while calendar year is a surrogate for nonspecific environmental exposures or secular changes in life-style factors.

Age at and Calendar Year of Hire

Modern industrial plants are generally much cleaner than those of yesteryear and thus the date of hire is often strongly correlated with exposure intensity. Differences in excess and relative risks according to age at hire are important in assessing whether the occupational exposure affects an early or late stage of the disease process (Day and Brown 1980).

Period of Employment

The "latent interval" is best defined in terms of excess disease risk as a function of time since initial employment, rather than from the observed distribution of time from employment to diagnosis in affected individuals (Peto 1985; Thomas 1987). The evolution of risk following the cessation of exposure may provide clues as to the nature of the disease process and has clear implications for public health policy. Gilbert (1982) demonstrated that short-term nuclear workers had elevated death rates, especially from infectious diseases, compared with more stable elements of the work force and also that death rates were higher in the years immediately following termination of employment. Both observations are presumably related to selection biases known collectively as the "healthy worker" effect.

Intensity of Exposure

Quantitative measurements of exposure in occupational studies are often based on the history of job titles and work areas and are thus subject to substantial errors that may bias the estimates of dose-response trends (B. Armstrong, this volume). Nevertheless, qualitative comparisons between workers of similar backgrounds who are employed in different parts of the plant is of great relevance because of the relative lack of selection and confounding bias.

Personal Characteristics

Differences between disease rates in the working cohort and those in the national or local comparison group are often ascribed to differences in ethnicity, education, social class and the personal habits that are correlated with these demographic variables. Moderate increases in lung cancer SMRs are essentially uninterpretable without concomitant information on smoking. A major issue in the statistical analysis of occupational cohort data is the control of confounding by personal characteristics for which data are lacking in the available company or union records (J. Spinelli, this volume).

Methods of Statistical Analysis

Person-Years and Rate Calculations

The first and often the most difficult step in the analysis of occupational cohort data is the categorization of each risk factor into discrete levels and the creation of a multidimensional table whose cells contain, for each combination of factor levels, the number of deaths from each cause of interest and the person-years of observation. Age and calendar year are usually included as factors and the product of standard rates by person-years thus gives the "expected" number of deaths as an additional cell entry for use in SMR analyses. When there are a large number of factors, the total number of cells can easily exceed the total number of observations. Many cells will contain no deaths and very few person-years of observation. (Those with no person-years need not be retained.) Nevertheless, construction of this table in as much detail as possible is recommended since it greatly facilitates the subsequent analyses. Computer programs are available for this purpose (Coleman et al. 1986; Marsh and Preininger 1980; Gilbert and Buchanan 1984; Preston and Pierce 1986; Waxweiler et al. 1983).

If interest is focused on a single time-dependent factor, the nonparametric estimate of the cumulative mortality rate (Nelson 1969) provides a powerful tool for descriptive analysis. Shore et al. (1977) used this to advantage in their study of breast cancer following radiation treatment for postpartum mastitis as did Peto et al. (1982) in their analysis of mesothelioma rates among asbestos insulation workers. Such exploratory analyses are highly recommended as a prelude to more formal inferential analyses.

A Single SMR for Each Cause of Death

In spite of its deficiencies, the usual table of SMRs by cause of death provides a useful synopsis of the relative effects of cohort membership on different diseases. It is wise to exclude the first few years of follow-up and to limit the calculation to members of the "stable" work force. The main point is not to stop here but to use this as a starting point for a more comprehensive analysis.

Within Cohort Comparison of SMRs

Current practice frequently involves the comparison of SMRs according to, for example, time since initial employment or predominant place of work. Formal statistical tests for heterogeneity and trend in such a series of SMRs are available. However, these are strictly valid only when the age/calendar year specific rates in each comparison group are a constant multiple of the standard rates and when the unexplained variation in SMRs is no more than that specified by the standard (Poisson) sampling assumptions. It is well known that comparison of indirectly standardized rates may be misleading when these conditions do not hold (Yule 1934; Miettinen 1972a). Examples are easily constructed where the trend in SMRs by exposure category points in the opposite direction from the trend in the age-specific rates. Closer examination reveals that the problem is one of confounding of the SMR ratios by age or calendar year and that it can be overcome by inclusion of the confounding variables in a carefully validated regression model (Breslow and Day 1985). However, this approach is tantamount to estimating the background rates internally.

Internal Standardization

Doll and colleagues (1970) attempted an adjusted analysis of individual risk factor effects by stratifying the sample on the remaining factors. The pooled stratum specific rates were then used as the "standard" to determine the expected numbers of deaths in each risk category in an SMR analysis. While it avoids some of the more extreme biases of comparisons based on an external standard, this approach is conservatively biased and the degree of conservatism increases with the degree of confounding between risk and control factors.

Mantel-Haenszel Analyses

The Mantel-Haenszel technique offers a simple, robust approach to summarizing the age/stratum specific rate ratios between two or more comparison groups (Rothman and Boice 1979). Related tests are available for testing the null hypothesis of equality in the age-specific rates against alternatives of heterogeneity or trend (Hakulinen 1981; Gilbert 1983). The Mantel-Haenszel methods do not suffer from the problems of SMR comparisons. Their main drawback is the limitation on the number of strata that affects any stratified analysis and the awkwardness of having to consider each risk factor separately rather than evaluating joint effects in a single comprehensive equation.

Poisson Regression Analysis of Grouped Cohort Data

Poisson regression analysis of the cross-classified numbers of deaths and person-years offers an efficient means of estimating the joint effects on mortality rates of several different risk factors (Holford 1980; Berry 1983; Frome 1983). Flexible computer programs like GLIM (Baker and Nelder 1978) and EGRET (Mauritsen 1988) facilitate the interactive fitting of many different models during a single work session. Incorporation of external standard rates into the model leads to a regression analysis of the SMR that can help identify situations where there is a serious problem of "noncomparability." Table 1 illustrates this aproach with grouped data from the Montana smelter workers study (Lee and Fraumeni 1969). The model with internal estimation of age- and calendar-year-specific respiratory cancer rates (not shown) yields estimated relative risks of approximately 1.6 for workers hired before 1925 vs those hired later and for foreign vs U.S. born and suggests an increase in rates according to the number of years of exposure especially to "high" levels of airborne arsenic. There is good agreement between the parameter estimates for this model and those for the SMR regression model in which calendar year has been included as a confounding variable.

Table 1. Regression coefficients estimated by the Poisson model for the Montana cohort. (From Breslow and Day 1987)

Variable	External SMR analysis Calendar year effects		Internal control
	Included	Excluded	
Constant	0.26	0.58	—
Hired before 1925	0.56	0.44	0.44
Foreign born	0.49	0.41	0.46
Heavy arsenic (years)			
1–4	0.17	0.20	0.19
5+	1.07	1.07	1.07
Moderate arsenic (years)			
1–4	0.59	0.60	0.60
5–14	0.25	0.26	0.26
15+	0.68	0.68	0.69
Calendar period			
1950–1959		−0.08	
1960–1969		−0.23	
1970–1977		−0.48	

Proportional Hazards Regression of Continuous Cohort Data

When the data are of sufficient magnitude and quality to justify a more refined approach, Cox's (1972) proportional hazards regression model provides for regression analysis of the data in their original continuous form. Two main differences with Poisson regression are: (a) the "Cox" model allows the baseline cumulative mortality rates associated with *one* of the time factors to be estimated nonparametrically; and (b) continuous, time-dependent covariables representing the entire past history of exposure may be incorporated into the regression equation. The price paid is a limitation on the possible model structures and greatly increased computing costs. Depending on the goals of the analysis, one may wish to use age, time since first employment, or time since entry into the cohort as the basic time variable in the analysis, with the effects of the other time factors being modeled parametrically. Caution is needed when controlling for time since first employment in this fashion lest one mask the very exposure effects one is looking for (Breslow et al. 1983).

Continuous time analyses of the SMR are accomplished by inserting the logarithm of the standard rates into the model equation as an *offset*, i.e., a time-dependent variable whose regression coefficient is fixed at unity (Andersen et al. 1985; Breslow and Langholz 1987). As an example, Fig. 1 presents smooth, nonparametric estimates of the SMR for respiratory cancer in the Montana study as a function of time since initial employment, with and without adjustment for covariates. After accounting for the strong effects of employment before 1925, when introduction of a selective flotation process markedly reduced airborne exposures, the apparent peak in the SMR some 30–40 years after employment completely disappears.

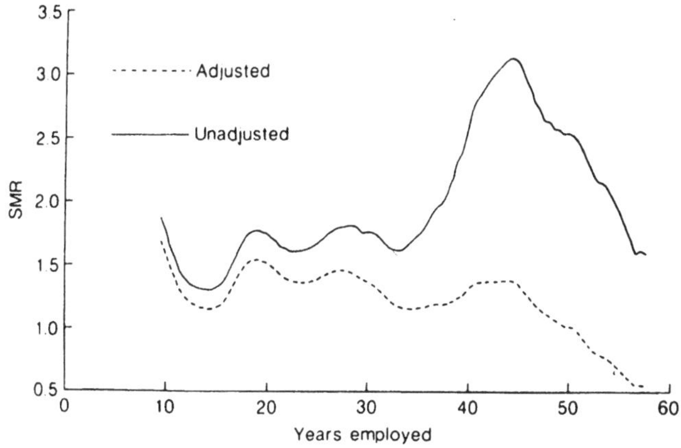

Fig. 1. Smoothed estimates of the standardized mortality ratio (SMR) for years since first employment for Montana smelter workers with (- - -) and without (———) adjustment for covariable effects. From Breslow and Langholz (1987)

Alternative Model Structures

Poisson regression is remarkably flexible in the variety of parametric model structures that it can accommodate. The computer program GLIM gives the user a choice between excess risk models in which the effects of different risk factors on disease rates combine additively, relative risk models in which the effects combine multiplicatively, and power law models in which a power transform of the rates is expressed as a linear combination of covariable effects. Maximum likelihood estimates of the best-fitting power transform are facilitated by GLIM macros that employ "constructed" regression variables based on the results of previous fits. Figure 2 graphs the deviances for a range of models fitted to coronary heart disease rates occurring among British doctors. Smoking neither adds a constant amount to the age-specific background rates, nor does it multiply them by a constant amount. Rather its effects are best expressed on an intermediate scale: smoking increases the square root of the background rates (cases per 1000 person-years) by half (Breslow and Day 1987).

As flexible as they are, one is by no means restricted to such "generalized linear models" with Poisson regression. Models with inherently nonlinear parameters are used increasingly (Frome 1983; Muirhead and Darby 1987). Preston and Pierce (1986) developed the computer program AMFIT to fit Poisson models where the rates are expressed as a sum of products of both linear and multiplicative functions of the regression variables. With continuous variable modelling, on the other hand, one is at present restricted to relative risk models for the covariable effects unless the baseline rates are estimated parametrically rather than nonparametrically.

A more ambitious approach to statistical modelling is to base the equation on an explicit biomathematical model of the disease process. For example, the

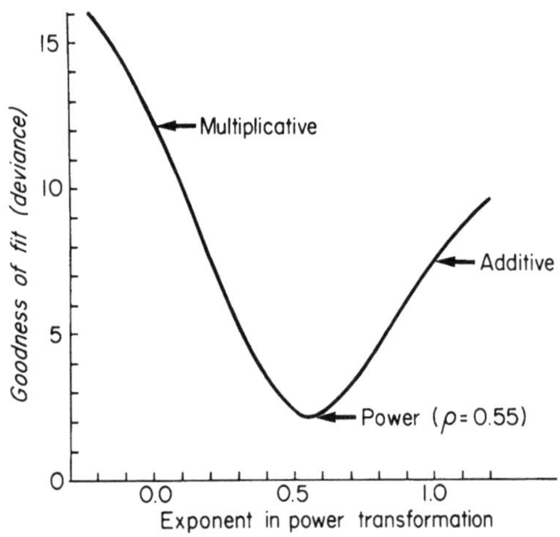

Fig. 2. Goodness-of fit statistics (deviances) for a variety of power models fitted to the British doctors data. From Breslow and Day (1987)

multistage model of carcinogenesis (Armitage and Doll 1961) predicts that a continuous lifetime exposure of constant intensity that affects exactly 2 of K stages will result in disease rates that are proportional to the square of the dose rate and the $K-1$ power of duration of exposure. Doll and Peto (1978) fitted this model to lung cancer data from the British doctors study grouped by smoking rate and age to arrive at the equation

$$\text{rate} = 0.273 \times 10^{-12}\ (\text{cigarettes/day} + 6)^2\ (\text{age} - 22.5)^{4.5}$$

for rates between 40 and 80 years of age. They argued that smokers tended to start smoking at about age 20–25 and that the exponent of 4.5 represented an (empirical) compromise between a disease process with 5 or 6 stages. Industrial exposures, however, are unlikely to occur at a constant rate over the lifespan and workers may vary substantially in the ages at which they start and stop exposure. Fitting of rather complicated dose-time-response models to the continuous data on exposure history is typically required in such circumstances. Thomas (1988) reviews a number of attempts that have been made to fit such models to epidemiological data.

Selection of Models and Variables

Criteria for the selection of a particular model equation include the plausibility of the basic model structure, the interpretability of the parameters in the model and the goodness-of-fit of the model to the data. When assessing the fit of any particular model, global measures such as the deviance or chi-square statistics should be supplemented by regression diagnostic procedures (Cook and Weisberg 1982) that identify particular regions of the data that are either poorly fit by the model or else have an inoridnate influence on the estimated parameters. The decision to engage in statistical modelling of any kind rests on the belief that the bias due to misspecification of the model structure is of lesser consequence than the reduction in variance from model-based estimates. More highly parameterized models lead to predictions of disease risk that are less biased by an inadequate model structure but more affected by sampling variability in the parameter estimates. Statisticians have suggested that goodness-of-fit measures such as the deviance be penalized by addition of twice the number of estimated parameters when evaluating models in terms of their ability to accurately predict future observations (Akaike 1973; Efron 1986). This criterion produces a reasonable tradeoff between bias and variance for models with varying numbers of parameters.

A notable deficiency in current statistical practice is the tendency to present results exclusively in terms of a single "best" model, chosen for example by a stepwise variable selection algorithm based upon some standard model form. This ignores the fact that other models that involve different variables or different structures, that have roughly equivalent explanatory power, and that fit the data equally well may have notably different epidemiologic interpretations or lead to notably different risk estimates, especially when these are extrapolated to or beyond the boundaries of the observed data. There is a much greater role for sensitivity analyses that explore the dependence of study conclusions on the modelling assumptions that are made in the course of the statistical analysis.

Collection and Analysis of Data on Personal Characteristics

A particular problem affecting occupational cohort studies is the fact that data on personal characteristics such as smoking, alcohol consumption and diet are not available in the usual industry records. Ascertainment of such covariable data may require expensive abstraction of medical charts or personal interviews. Several proposals have been made to limit the number of subjects for whom covariable data need to be collected and analyzed.

Nested Case-Control Studies

Analysis of cohort data via the proportional hazards model involves the enumeration of the distinct times at which the events of interest occur and the formation of risk sets consisting of all subjects who were under observation just prior to that time. Regression variables of the cases in each risk set are compared with those of the non-cases using a probability model in which the conditional probability of being a case is assumed proportional to the relative risk. The number of risk sets is typically small in comparison with the number of subjects and can be reduced even further by minor grouping of observations along the time axis. For example, in our analyses of the 8014 Montana smelter workers followed between 1938 and 1963 the 142 respiratory cancer deaths gave rise to 91 distinct risk sets defined by integral ages (in years) and 5-year calendar periods at death. Since the average risk set size was 322 subjects, this effectively meant that 30 000 data records needed to be processed for each iteration in the fitting algorithm. Thomas (1977) suggested that one could approximate the resultant estimates by drawing a small sample of control subjects, usually no more than four or five, from each risk set and performing the same analysis on reduced risk sets consisting of just the cases and sampled controls. For the Montana study, this would reduce the number of subjects for whom covariable data needed to be collected from 8000 to about 450 (or fewer, since some controls may be sampled in more than one risk set). Similarly it would reduce the effective size of the data file needed for the full analysis from 30 000 to 450. Table 2 demonstrates that the nested case-control approach accomplished its goal of approximating the results of the full proportional hazards analysis (Breslow et al. 1983). However, more than four or five controls per risk set may be desirable when the object is to accurately approximate the relative risks associated with rare exposures and the cost of additional data collection is not at issue.

Table 2. Comparison of regression coefficients and standard errors from Cox regression analysis of Montana data with those from nested case-control samples. (From Breslow et al. 1983)

Variable	Cox model	Nested case-control $n=20$	$n=10$	$n=5$
	A. Regression coefficients			
Foreign born	0.72	0.70	0.66	0.75
No. of decades of heavy arsenic exposure	0.60	0.69	0.74	0.85
No. of decades of moderate arsenic exposure	0.22	0.21	0.29	0.35
	B. Standard errors			
Foreign born	0.20	0.21	0.23	0.25
No. of decades of heavy arsenic exposure	0.13	0.16	0.18	0.23
No. of decades of moderate arsenic exposure	0.07	0.08	0.10	0.11

Case-Cohort Sampling

Prentice (1986) proposed an alternative case-cohort design for use especially with disease prevention trials where all subjects are enrolled during the same short calendar period. A subcohort is sampled at the outset for purposes of covariable ascertainment and analysis. As disease cases occur outside this subcohort, additional covariable data are collected for them. Risk sets are formed from the pool of subcohort members plus other cases and the analysis proceeds as before. However, estimation of the standard errors of the regression coefficients is more complicated due to the necessity of accounting for correlations between risk set contributions to the (pseudo) likelihood equations.

The case-cohort design appears more advantageous than the nested case-control design for two reasons. First, when more than one disease outcome is to be considered, controls in the single subcohort may be compared with the cases of each disease. A completely separate control sample would be required for each disease with the nested case-control approach. Second, since subcohort members and cases are analyzed in each risk set in which they occur, whereas controls in the nested study are analyzed only in the particular risk sets from which they were sampled, the risk set sizes for the case-cohort study tend to be larger for the same total number of subjects and standard errors of the parameter estimates are accordingly smaller. However, Langholz and Thomas (unpublished data) have shown that this improvement in efficiency is not nearly so great as imagined earlier due to the fact that controls may be sampled more than once with the nested design. Furthermore, when the entry period is spread widely over calendar time and there is considerable censoring due to deaths from competing causes or loss-to-follow-up, the case-cohort design loses efficiency because the latest risk sets contain too few controls.

Two-Stage Designs

A serious drawback to both the nested case-control and case-cohort designs is that they ignore data on exposure and disease for subjects not included in the subsamples selected for covariable ascertainment. If exposure is rare, both may fail to sample many of the informative subjects who are exposed and disease-free. One needs "selectivity in both series" so that all rare subjects, whether cases or exposed, are included in the sample (Miettinen 1972b).

A "two-stage" design is now available that accomplishes this goal. At the conclusion of the cohort study, subjects are classified jointly on the basis of the disease outcome and a small number of exposure categories. Balanced subsamples consisting of an equal number of cases and controls are drawn from each exposure stratum for purposes of covariable ascertainment. When both the exposure indicator and the covariable are binary, White (1982) demonstrated how to combine the data from both first and second stage samples to estimate a covariable adjusted relative risk with appropriate standard error. Breslow and Cain (1988) developed the requisite modifications of logistic regression analysis so that the design could be used also with multiple or continuous variables. When a separate relative risk is to be estimated for each of the exposure strata used to select the second stage sample, simple adjustments are made to the logistic analysis of the second stage data so as to correct the regression coefficients for the biased sampling and their standard errors for the extra information available in the first stage data.

The two-stage design is illustrated here with data from the first 18 years of the Framingham study (Kannél and Gordon 1974). Table 3 shows the distribution of 5052 study subjects with no prior diagnosis of coronary heart disease (CHD) who had known values for the relevant baseline covariables. From each of the

Table 3. Distribution of 5052 Framingham residents by age, sex, and CHD. (First 18 years of FU)

Age	Males		Females	
(years)	CHD	No CHD	CHD	No CHD
30–39	73	742	24	996
40–49	158	603	75	870
50+	189	481	154	687
Total	420	1826	253	2553

Table 4. Regression coefficients and standard errors in logistic analysis of CHD risk in Framingham

Variable	Full dataset ($n=5052$)	Balanced sample ($n=298$)	
		Unadjusted	Adjusted
A) Regression coefficients			
Constant	−1.42	−0.18	−1.28
Sex	−0.85	0.14	−0.92
Age	0.68	−0.14	0.68
FRW	0.95	−0.12	−0.07
SBP	1.56	2.58	2.55
Cigarettes	0.38	0.26	0.27
B) Standard errors			
Constant	0.10	0.23	0.16
Sex	0.10	0.26	0.16
Age	0.06	0.16	0.11
FRW	0.27	0.78	0.78
SBP	0.18	0.61	0.62
Cigarettes	0.07	0.23	0.23

FRW, Framingham relative weight; SBP, systolic blood pressure.

six age/sex strata, 25 cases who developed CHD and 25 controls were sampled, except that for females aged 30–39 years all 24 available cases and an equal number of controls were used. Table 4 presents the results of logistic regression analyses for the entire cohort of 5052 subjects and for the sample of 248 subjects, with and without appropriate adjustment for the known sampling ratios. Adjustment is needed to get unbiased estimates of the coefficients for age and sex. The difference between adjusted and unadjusted standard errors shows how much the use of the first stage data improves the precision. Note that the coefficients and standard errors for the "covariables" Framingham relative weight, systolic blood pressure and cigarettes are little affected by the adjustment since most of the information about them comes from the subsamples.

Dealing with Selection Bias; the Healthy Worker Effect

Perhaps the most difficult issue to deal with in the statistical analysis of occupational cohort data is "healthy worker" selection bias. Persons selected for initial employment tend to have lower mortality rates than the general population, and those who remain at work many years later have lower mortality rates than those who have already terminated (Fox and Collier 1976). Workers who accumulate the heaviest exposures tend to be those who have worked the longest and stayed the healthiest. Peto (1985) has called attention to the dose-response fallacy that results from uncritical examination of relative or excess risks according to categories of cumulative exposure. Mortality rates are generally lower during the first few years following entry into a new cumulative exposure category by virtue of the fact that a person is necessarily still employed at the time of crossing the boundary. This biases the dose-response curve in the direction of a negative relationship.

The essential dilemma here is the existence of an unmeasured confounding variable, namely health status, that strongly affects both continuing exposure and disease mortality. Workers who develop signs or symptoms of chronic illness, even before an outright diagnosis, are removed from hazardous areas or voluntarily terminate their employment and thus cease their exposure. Gilbert (1983) suggested lagging the time-dependent exposure variables by a period of 2 or more years on the grounds that: (a) any exposure received within, say, 2 years of death could not have contributed to it; and (b) the disease process is so rapid that signs or symptoms would not appear earlier than 2 years prior to death and so could not influence exposure during that period. These assumptions seem reasonable for a disease like lung cancer that has a long latent interval and a rapidly fatal course. However, they do not apply when the endpoint is cardiovascular disease mortality. Robins (1987) has proposed some rather complicated analytic procedures for this situation whose validity also, unfortunately, rests on untestable assumptions. Nonetheless, some further experience with his proposals would be desirable.

Conclusions

Statistical methods for the analysis of occupational cohort data are now available that make full use of the collected data and that avoid some of the more obvious biases associated with traditional SMR analyses. Nonparametric estimates of cumulative mortality rates and ratios as a function of age and other time variables lend themselves to exploratory, graphical analyses as a prelude to formal model building. Poisson regression analyses of multidimensional tables of deaths and person-years make efficient use of the data and are flexible as regards model structure. Proportional hazards analyses of continuous data are available for special situations. Provided that appropriate regression analyses are carried out to validate their use, tables of observed and expected numbers of deaths by various combinations of exposure factors offer a convenient way of summarizing the results of the study in synoptic form for publication. Several new methods of design and analysis of substudies of covariable effects should see increasing use in future years. Lagged exposure variables provide one means, admittedly imperfect, of dealing with “healthy worker” selection biases.

References

Akaike H (1973) Information theory and an extension of the maximum likelihood principle. In: Petrov BN, Czaki F (eds) Second international symposium on information theory. Akademiac Kiado, Budapest, pp 267–281

Andersen PK, Borch-Johnsen K, Deckert T, Green A, Hougoard P, Keiding N, Kreiner S (1985) A Cox regression model for the relative mortality and its application to diabetes mellitus survival data. Biometrics 41: 921–932

Armitage P, Doll R (1961) Stochastic models for carcinogenesis. In: Proceedings of the 4th Berkeley Symposium on mathematical statistics and probability: biology and problems of health. University of California Press, Berkeley, pp 19–38

Baker RJ, Nelder JA (1978) The GLIM system: release 3. Numerical Algorithms Group, Oxford

Berry G (1983) The analysis of mortality by the subject-years method. Biometrics 39: 173–184

Breslow NE, Cain KC (1988) Logistic regression for two-stage case-control data. Biometrika 75: 11–20

Breslow NE, Day NE (1985) The standardized mortality ratio. In: Sen PK, (ed) Biostatistics: statistics in biomedical, public health and environmental sciences. Elsevier, New York, pp 55–74

Breslow NE, Day NE (1987) Statistical methods in cancer research II: design and analysis of cohort studies. International Agency for Research on Cancer, Lyon

Breslow NE, Langholz B (1987) Nonparametric estimation of relative mortality functions. J Chronic Dis 40 [Suppl 2]: 895–995

Breslow NE, Lubin JH, Marek P, Langholz B (1983) Multiplicative models and cohort analysis. J Am Stat Assoc 78: 1–12

Cochran WG (1983) Planning and analysis of observational studies. Wiley, New York

Coleman M, Douglas A, Hermon C, Peto J (1986) Cohort study analysis with a FORTRAN computer program. Int J Epidemiol 15: 134–137

Cook RD, Weisberg S (1982) Residuals and influence in regression. Chapman and Hall, London

Cox DR (1972) Regression models and life tables (with discussion). J R Stat Soc B 34: 187–220

Day NE, Brown CC (1980) Multistage models and the primary prevention of cancer. J NCI 64: 977–989

Doll R, Peto R (1978) Cigarette smoking and bronchial carcinoma: dose and time relationships among regular smokers and life-long non-smokers. J Epidemiol Community Health 32: 303–313

Doll R, Morgan LG, Speizer F (1970) Cancers of the lung and nasal sinuses in nickel workers. Br J Cancer 24: 623–632

Efron B (1986) How biased is the apparent error rate of a prediction rule? J Am Stat Assoc 81: 461–470

Fox AJ, Collier PF (1976) Low mortality rates in industrial cohort studies due to selection for work and survival in the industry. Br J Prev Soc Med 30: 225–230

Frome EL (1983) The analysis of rates using Poisson regression models. Biometrics 39: 665–674

Gaffey WR (1976) A critique of the standardized mortality ratio. J Occup Med 18: 157–160

Gardner MR (1986) Considerations in the choice of expected numbers of appropriate comparisons in occupational cohort studies. Med Law 77: 23–47
Gilbert ES (1982) Some confounding factors in the study of mortality and occupational exposures. Am J Epidemiol 116: 177–188
Gilbert ES (1983) An evaluation of several methods for assessing the effects of occupational exposure to radiation. Biometrics 39: 161–171
Gilbert ES, Buchanan JA (1984) An alternative approach to analyzing occupational mortality data. J Occup Med 11: 822–828
Hakulinen T (1981) A Mantel-Haenszel statistic for testing the association between a polychotomous exposure and a rare outcome. Am J Epidemiol 113: 192–197
Hill AB (1953) Observation and experiment. N Engl J Med 248: 995–1001
Holford TR (1980) The analysis of rates and of survivorship using log-linear models. Biometrics 36: 229–306
Kannel WB, Gordon T (1974) The Framingham study. US Government Printing Office, Washington (DHEW publ no (NIH) 74–559)
Lee AM, Fraumeni JF Jr (1969) Arsenic and respiratory cancer in man: an occupational study. J NCI 42: 1045–1052
Marsh GM, Preininger ME (1980) OCCMAP: a user-oriented occupational cohort mortality analysis program. Am Statist 34: 245–246
Mauritsen RH (1988) EGRET manual. Statistics and Epidemiology Research Corporation, Seattle
Miettinen OS (1972a) Standardization of risk ratios. Am J Epidemiol 96: 383–388
Miettinen OS (1972b) Design options in epidemiologic research: an update. Scand J Work Environ Health 8 [Suppl 1]: 7–14
Muirhead CR, Darby SC (1987) Modelling the relative and absolute risks of radiation-induced cancers (with discussion). J R Stat Soc A 150: 83–118
Nelson W (1969) Hazard plotting for incomplete failure data. J Quality Technol 1: 27–52
Peto J (1985) Some problems in dose-response estimation in cancer epidemiology. In: Voug VB, Butler GB, Hoel DG, Peakall DB (eds) Methods for estimating risk of chemical injury: human and non-human biota and ecosystems. Wiley, New York, pp 361–380
Peto J, Seidman H, Selikoff IJ (1982) Mesothelioma mortality in asbestos workers: implications for models of carcinogenesis and risk. Br J Cancer 45: 124–135
Prentice RL (1986) A case-cohort design for epidemiologic cohort studies and disease prevention trials. Biometrika 73: 1–12
Preston DL, Pierce DA (1986) Program documentation for AMFIT and PYTABS. Radiation Effects Research Foundation, Hiroshima
Robins J (1987) A graphical approach to the identification and estimation of causal parameters in mortality studies with sustained exposure periods. J Chronic Dis 40 [Suppl 2]: 1395–1615
Rothman KJ, Boice JD Jr (1979) Epidemiologic analysis with a programmable calculator. US Government Printing Office, Washington (NIH publ no 79–1649)
Saracci R, Johnson E (1987) A note on the treatment of time in published cancer epidemiology studies. J Chronic Dis 40 [Suppl 2]: 77S–78S
Shore RE, Hempelmann LH, Kowaluk E, Mansur PS, Pasternack BS, Albert RE, Haughie GE (1977) Breast neoplasms in women treated with x-rays for acute postpartum mastitis. J NCI 59: 813–822
Thomas DC (1977) Addendum to a paper by Liddell FDK, McDonald JC, Thomas DC. J R Stat Soc A 140: 483–485

Thomas DC (1987) Pitfalls in the analysis of exposure-time-response relationships. J Chronic Dis 40 [Suppl 2]: 71S–78S

Thomas DC (1988) Models for exposure-time-response relationships with applications to cancer epidemiology. Annu Rev Public Health 9: 451–482

Waxweiler RJ et al. (1983) A modified life-table analysis system for cohort studies. J Occup Med 25(2): 115–124

White JE (1982) A two stage design for the study of the relationship between a rare exposure and a rare disease. Am J Epidemiol 115: 119–128

Yule GU (1934) On some points relating to vital statistics, more especially statistics of occupational mortality. J R Stat Soc 97: 1–84

*Towards an Automated Micronucleus Assay as an Internal Dosimeter for Carcinogen-Exposed Human Population Groups**

H.F. Stich, A.B. Acton, and B. Palcic

Environmental Carcinogenesis Unit, and Cancer Imaging Section, British Columbia Cancer Research Centre, 601 West 10th Avenue, Vancouver, B.C. V5Z 1L3, Canada

Introduction

Predictions concerning human responses to carcinogen exposures depend to a large extent on the extrapolation of results obtained from tissue cultures or animal models. Because of differences in the pharmacology of carcinogens in different species, such extrapolations are of restricted value. Furthermore, there is a tendency to compare the effects of high carcinogen doses such as are used in experiments with cultured cells and rodents, with the actions of low doses to which humans are usually exposed. These difficulties can be overcome by using markers which are applicable to cultured cells, animal models and human subjects. We have previously shown that micronuclei are suitable internal dosimeters for revealing tissue-specific genotoxic damage in individuals exposed to carcinogenic mixtures (Stich et al. 1982a, b; Stich 1987; Stich and Rosin 1983, 1985) and for following the response to chemopreventive agents in short-term intervention trials (Stich 1986a, b, 1987; Stich et al. 1984, 1988). In this paper, we place particular emphasis on the automated scoring of micronuclei, which would make this test applicable to large-scale studies of human population groups.

Micronuclei: Background and Definition

Micronuclei have recently received considerable attention. As examples, they have been used as markers in genotoxic tests for carcinogens (Bruce and Heddle 1979; Jenssen and Ramel 1980; Schlegel and MacGregor 1984), in detecting organ-specific effects of carcinogens in animals (Wargovich et al. 1983; Blakey et al. 1985; Ronen and Heddle 1984), in tracing the transplacental action of genotoxic agents (Cole et al. 1981; Henderson et al. 1984), in examining the

* This study was supported by a grant from the National Cancer Institute of Canada. Dr. H.F. Stich is a Terry Fox Cancer Research Scientist of the National Cancer Institute of Canada.

Recent Results in Cancer Research, Vol. 120

effect of protein deficiency (Rabello-Gay et al. 1985), in quantitating the synergistic actions of smoking and alcohol consumption (Stich and Rosin 1983), in recognizing patients with chromosomal instability syndromes (Rosin and German 1985; Rosin and Ochs 1986), in identifying carcinogen-exposed human tissues at elevated risk for cancer (Raafat et al. 1984; Stich and Rosin 1985; Mandard et al. 1987), in the prognosis of nonlymphocytic leukaemia (Högstedt et al. 1981), in evaluating the response to antileukaemic agents (Abe et al. 1984), and in following the response to the administration of chemopreventive agents in clinical trials (Stich et al. 1984, 1985).

The term "micronucleus" has been applied to a variety of structures, all of which give a positive Feulgen reaction, are located in the cytoplasm, have no connection to the main cell nucleus, and are considerably smaller than the main nucleus. Micronuclei result from acentric chromosome and chromatid fragments or from aberrant chromosomes which have not been included in the main nucleus, and thus appear as separate entities in the cytoplasm. Our recent electron microscopic studies have revealed numerous small micronuclei which would escape detection in a light microscopic examination (Figs. 1–6). Furthermore, the tiny Feulgen-positive, irregular, round clumps seen by light microscopy also proved to be membrane-bound micronuclei containing internal structures which resemble chromatin (Figs. 1 and 2). Many investigators exclude irregularly shaped cytoplasmic DNA bodies from their micronuclei counts. In our laboratory, we score all Feulgen-positive bodies because of the difficulty in distinguishing one micronucleus from another. Thus, our scores of micronucleated cells are somewhat higher than those of, for example, Fontham et al. (1986) and Munoz et al. (1987), who restrict their counts to the larger round bodies in the cytoplasm.

If the size distribution of the micronuclei follows a fixed pattern, then whether all Feulgen-positive bodies are served, or only the larger ones that can be positively identified as round, membrane-bound micronuclei under the light microscope, should not affect the comparison between controls and carcinogen-exposed tissues. However, the question must be asked whether the size distribution of micronuclei actually varies in cell populations exposed to different doses of one genotoxic agent, or among cells treated with different genotoxic chemicals. To resolve this issue we measured the sizes of micronuclei in Chinese hamster ovary (CHO) cells exposed for 3 h to methyl methanesulfonate (MMS) and benzo(a)pyrene (B(a)P), respectively. No major differences in the size distribution pattern were detected between two different doses of MMS or between MMS and B(a)P treatment (Fig. 7). However, a completely different distribution pattern became evident when the effect of a chromatid-breaking agent (MMS) was compared with that of colchicine which blocks the formation of mitotic spindles and leads to aberrant chromosomes (Fig. 8). The results clearly show that large micronuclei predominate in the colchicine-treated cell population. Thus, a comparative study that would restrict the scoring to only the large bodies could lead to erroneous conclusions. We suggest that all detectable DNA-positive micronuclei should be scored, and that no arbitrary

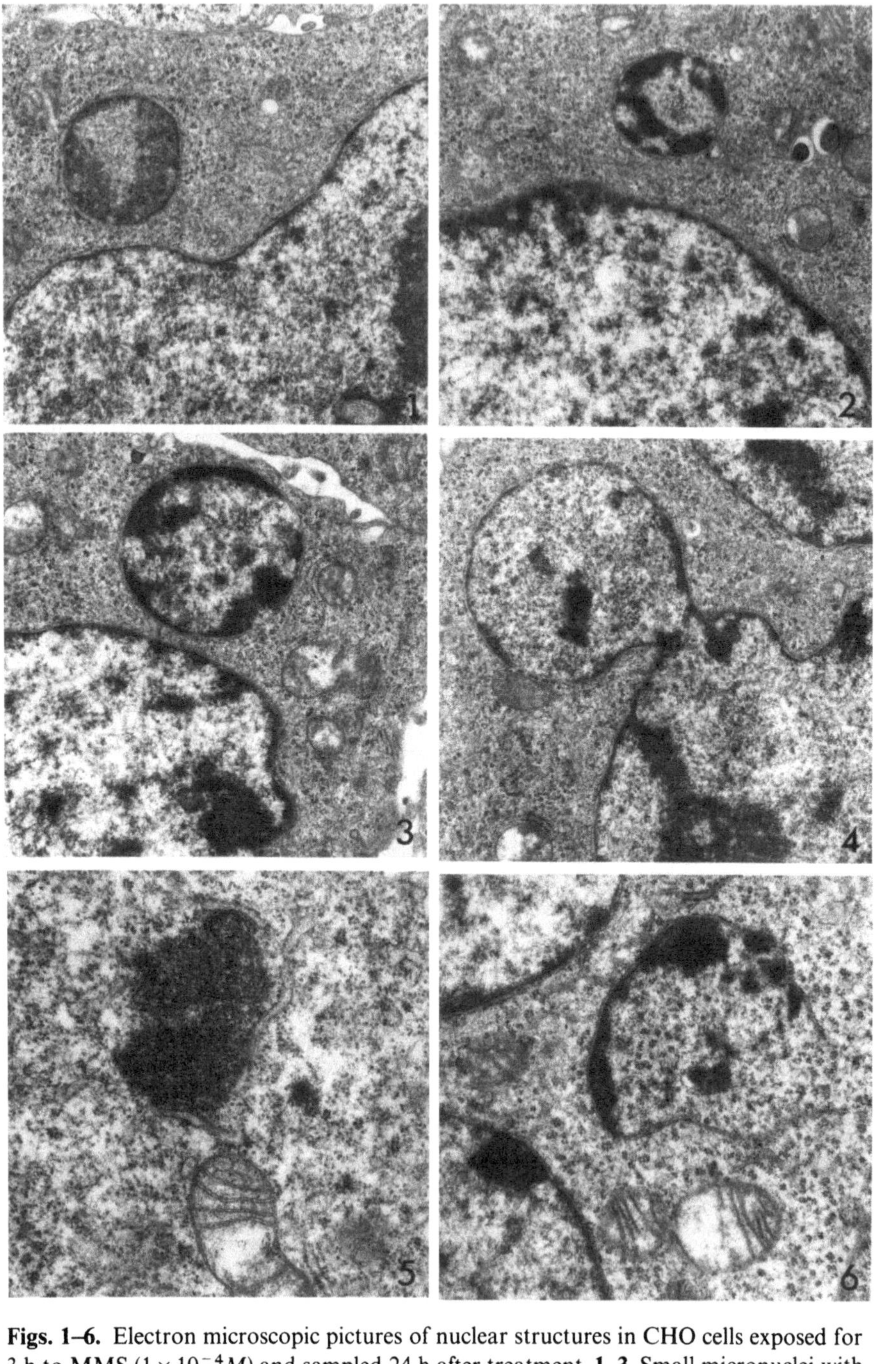

Figs. 1–6. Electron microscopic pictures of nuclear structures in CHO cells exposed for 3 h to MMS ($1 \times 10^{-4} M$) and sampled 24 h after treatment. **1–3** Small micronuclei with nuclear membranes and internal structures. **4** Nuclear protrusion which, on light microscopic examination, could be mistaken for a micronucleus. **5** A chromatid or chromosome fragment which is partially surrounded by a nuclear membrane. This structure will later form a micronucleus. **6** Micronucleus into which cytoplasmic components are being included.

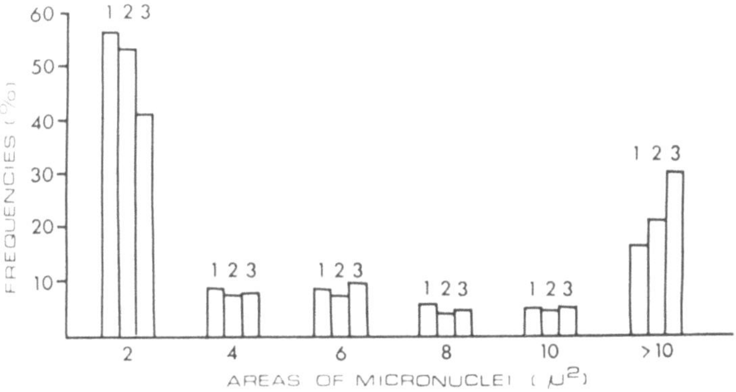

Fig. 7. Size distribution of micronuclei in CHO cells exposed for 3 h to (*1*) MMS at $1 \times 10^{-4} M$ ($n=761$) or (*2*) $4 \times 10^{-4} M$ ($n=708$) and (*3*) B (a) P at $5 \times 10^{-4} M$ ($n=468$), and sampled 24 h after treatment (Feulgen reaction measurements done visually on enlarged photographs)

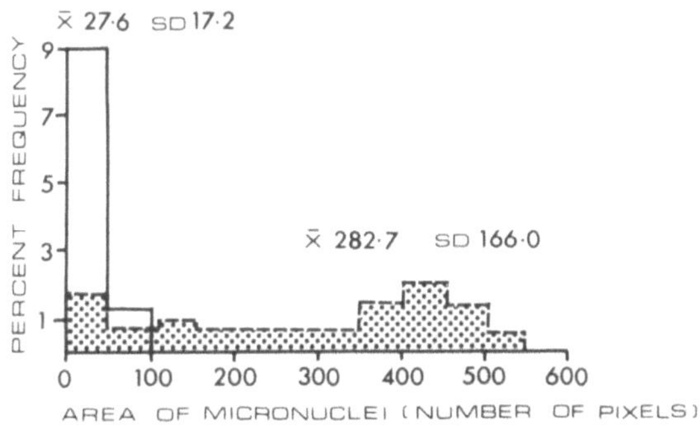

Fig. 8. Different size distribution of micronuclei in CHO cells treated with the mutagenic MMS ($1 \times 10^{-4} M$, *lined boxes*) and the spindle toxin colchicine (final concentration 0.001%, *dotted boxes*) for 3 h (Feulgen reaction, image analysis)

line should be drawn between small and large Feulgen-positive structures in the cytoplasm.

Micronuclei as Internal Dosimeters

A measure of the range of biologically effective doses of carcinogens in various human tissues would be highly desirable. However, prior to accepting micronuclei as internal markers, several issues must be resolved. Among them the collection of human specimens appears to be of primary importance. Exfoliated cells can be readily obtained from oral and nasal mucosa, sputum and urine using noninvasive procedures. In these cases, repeated sampling is feasible. This possibility is a prerequisite when responses to the administration of chemo-preventive agents are being traced, when the progression of precancerous lesions into carcinomas is being followed and when the efficacy of chemotherapeutic agents is being evaluated. On the other hand, the collection of exfoliated cells from cervical, oesophageal and bronchial tissues is semi-invasive, and can be repeated only at longer time intervals. Another approach consists of scoring micronuclei in tissue sections. However, since the taking of biopsy material is in most cases restricted to diagnostic or therapeutic purposes, this approach is not acceptable for large-scale population studies. Somewhat neglected are the immense possibilities offered for study by human tissue sections and smears which are stored in pathology departments around the globe. By using this material, the frequency of micronucleated cells can be traced throughout the medical history of a patient.

A possible source of error is the variation in the site from which exfoliated cells are sampled, since the frequency of micronuclei can vary among different areas of a carcinogen-exposed tissue (Stich 1987). For example, the highest frequency of micronucleated cells was observed in areas of the oral mucosa which come into close contact with betel quids or snuff (Stich et al. 1982b; Stich 1987). Brushings, swabbings, or flushings of large tissue regions will invariably contain a mixture of cells from areas with high and low frequencies of micronucleated cells. This "averaging" of the counts could result in an under- or overestimation of the real frequency of micronucleated cells in a particular tissue segment. Moreover, frequencies of micronuclei could be affected by the mistaken inclusion of individuals with chromosome instability syndromes (Rosin and Ochs 1986) into the "control" group. The sampling of tissues infected by viruses that produce chromosome aberrations (Stich and Yohn 1970) could also elevate the formation of micronuclei in "controls".

A further complication of the micronucleus assay is the necessity of cells to divide. Chromatid and chromosome fragments or aberrant chromosomes can only be excluded from a nucleus during mitosis. Thus, differences in the mitotic rate of various cell populations could affect the scoring of micronucleated cells and lead to erroneous conclusions. There are several ways to cope with this situation. Micronuclei in tissues with similar mitotic rates are directly comparable. The mitotic rate can be readily estimated on biopsy specimens which are either treated in organ cultures with colchicine to accumulate metaphases or with H^3TdR to measure DNA synthesis. A more convenient procedure is to restrict the scoring procedure to binucleated cells which can occur "spontaneously", or are induced by the application of cytochalasin-B which in the lymphocyte system proved to be the method of choice (Fenech and Morley 1985a, b, 1986).

A more detailed discussion of the pros and cons of the micronucleus test can be found in a previous publication (Stich 1987). If we consider that the micronucleus assay has only recently been applied to human tissues, then the results on human population groups that are exposed to environmental or lifestyle carcinogens or carcinogenic mixtures are quite impressive (Table 1).

Table 1. Frequency of micronuclei in human tissues at elevated risk for cancer

Tissue	Suspected carcinogenic factors	Elevation of micronucleated cells (fold)	Reference
Oral mucosa:			
Gingival groove	Snuff	4.2	Stich et al. (1985)
Inner lip	Khaini tobacco	4.4	Stich et al. (1982a)
Floor of mouth	Nass	8.2	Stich (1987)
Buccal mucosa	Betel quid	9.4	Stich et al. (1982b)
	Smoking and drinking	4.6	Stich and Rosin (1983)
	Smoking	3.4	Fontham et al. (1986)
	Curry	1.5	Picker and Fox (1986)
Oesophagus	Unknown (oesophagitis)	3.4	H.F. Stich and D.G. Zaridze (unpublished data)
	Smoking	[a]	Mandard et al. (1987)
Urinary bladder	*Schistosoma haematobium*	13.5	Raafat et al. (1984)
	Smoking	6.0	Fontham et al. (1986)
	Smoking and coffee drinking	9.4	Stich (1987)
	Smoking	Shift to higher values	Reali et al. (1987)
Bronchial epithelium	Smoking	2.6	Fontham et al. (1986)
	Smoking	2.2	H.F. Stich (unpublished data)
Cervical epithelium	Smoking	5.1	Fontham et al. (1986)
	Unknown (dysplasia)	3.0	Stich (1987)
Blood lymphocytes	Styrene	1.5	Högstedt et al. (1983)
	Styrene	9.0	Meretoja et al. (1978)
	Styrene	4.0	Nordenson and Beckman (1984)
	X-ray contrast media	1.6–4.3	Parvez et al. (1987)
Bone marrow	Antileukaemic agents	> 34.0	Abe et al. (1984)
Spermatids	Smoking	1.4	Lähdetie (1986)

[a] Elevated frequencies were observed in only 5% of patients examined.

Micronuclei in Chemopreventive Trials

A considerable number of studies have been dedicated to the search for so-called intermediate endpoints, which could predict the development of pre-cancerous lesions. These endpoints are envisaged as surrogates for cancer. Since micronuclei can reveal exposure levels of a tissue to carcinogens, and since the incidence of cancer is linked to exposure levels of carcinogens, the use of this cell marker seems to be justified. Based on this assumption, the micronucleus assay was recently applied to follow the response of tobacco chewers to the administration of chemopreventive agents. A reduction in the frequency of micronucleated cells following the administration of chemopreventive agents should indicate the efficacy of these agents in preventing carcinogen-induced injury to the genome. The rationale of this approach is also based on the hypothesis that an increase in micronuclei indicates a reshuffling of gene sequences, including oncogenes, and that this will increase the chance of neoplastic transformation. Consequently, a reduction in the frequency of micronuclei will diminish the probability of a genomic reshuffling. Our recent pilot intervention trials were conducted on fishermen in Kerala (India), who chewed an average of 17 betel quids daily and are at elevated risk for oral carcinomas. The chewers were distributed at random into four groups: I, placebo capsules; II, beta-carotene (180 mg/week); III, beta-carotene (180 mg/week) plus vitamin A (100 000 IU/week); and IV, vitamin A (200 000 IU/week). The participants continued to chew in their accustomed manner during the entire course of the trial. All treatments led to a reduction in the number of micronucleated cells, to a remission of oral leucoplakias, and to a reduced development of new leucoplakias. Figure 9 shows the rapid reduction in micronucleated buccal mucosa cells and the slower remission of oral leucoplakias among chewers receiving beta-carotene and vitamin A.

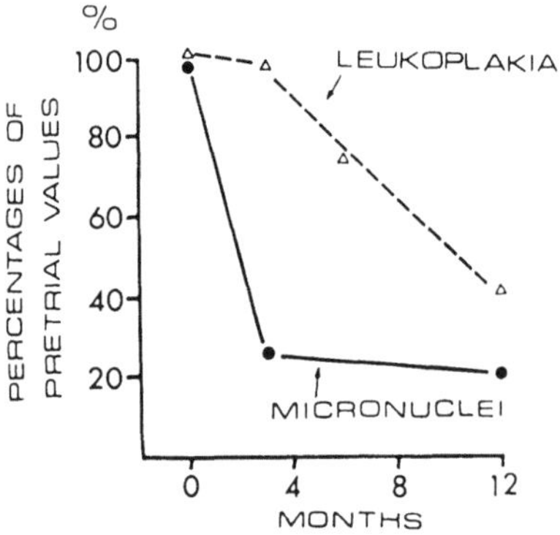

Fig. 9. Reduction of micronucleated oral mucosa cells and concomitant remission of oral leucoplakia during an intervention trial with beta-carotene on tobacco/betel nut chewers

Automated Detection of Micronuclei

To detect small but significant changes in the frequency of micronucleated cells, relatively large numbers of micronuclei must be scored. Assuming a 1% to 2% background frequency of micronucleated cells, it would require the examination of 500 to 2000 cells to detect a two-fold increase within a 95% confidence interval. Assaying such a large number of cells is tedious, slow and expensive. It is also open to subjective interpretations. Thus, if the micronucleus assay should become routinely used as a diagnostic tool or should become applicable to monitor larger population groups, it must be fully automated.

An automated scoring system requires the preparation of stained cells (e.g., Feulgen reaction or the fluorochrome Hoechst 33258) (MacGregor et al. 1983) with a minimum of overlap to minimize the incidence of false positive and negative errors. Such a scoring system must (a) discriminate between nuclear and cytoplasmic material; (b) recognize fully separated micronuclei from main nuclei (Fig. 10); (c) recognize partially separated (touching) micronuclei from main nuclei (Fig. 10); (d) measure area of nucleus and micronucleus; (e) measure DNA content of nucleus and micronucleus; (f) measure shape parameters of nucleus and micronucleus; (g) measure texture parameters (distribution) of DNA in the nucleus and micronucleus; and (h) mark nuclei of cells

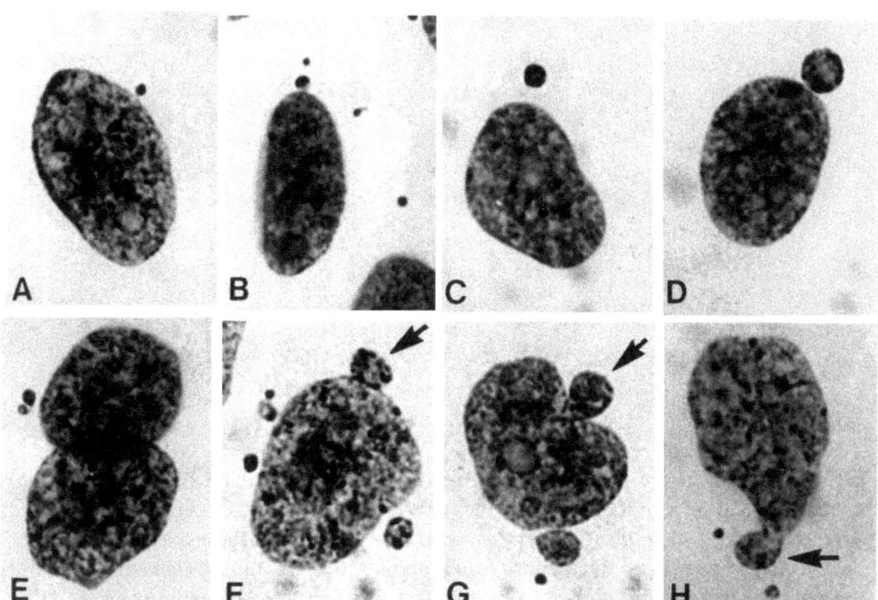

Fig. 10 A–H. Various shapes and sizes of micronuclei found in CHO cells exposed for 3 h to MMS ($1 \times 10^{-4} M$). *Arrows* point to structures which could be either micronuclei or nuclear protrusions

which divided at least once prior to sampling (binucleated cells) (Fenech and Morley 1986).

Due to the small size of most micronuclei, a high spatial resolution will be required. This calls for a good optical resolution with available sensors. Precise segmentation of nuclear material from the cytoplasm will require a high degree of spectral resolution, particularly as the segmentation has to be made fast and reliable. For estimating the amount of DNA in nuclei and micronuclei, including very small ones, a very high photometric resolution must be achieved. In many cases, fluorescent nuclear stain may prove more advantageous than conventional stoichiometric nuclear stains.

At present, there is no image cytometry device commercially available which would fulfill all the above requirements (Callisen et al. 1986). We believe that the development of such a system is possible. However, it would require a new generation of image cytometry devices. The present-day image cytometry devices have been designed by equipping a conventional microscope with an image transducer, most often a video tube. Neither the optical properties of the microscope, nor the sensing properties of the video transducers are adequate for the development of a simple and inexpensive apparatus for micronucleus detection and characterization in a fast and reliable manner. All the above-listed objectives can be met by a Solid State Microscope, which is currently under

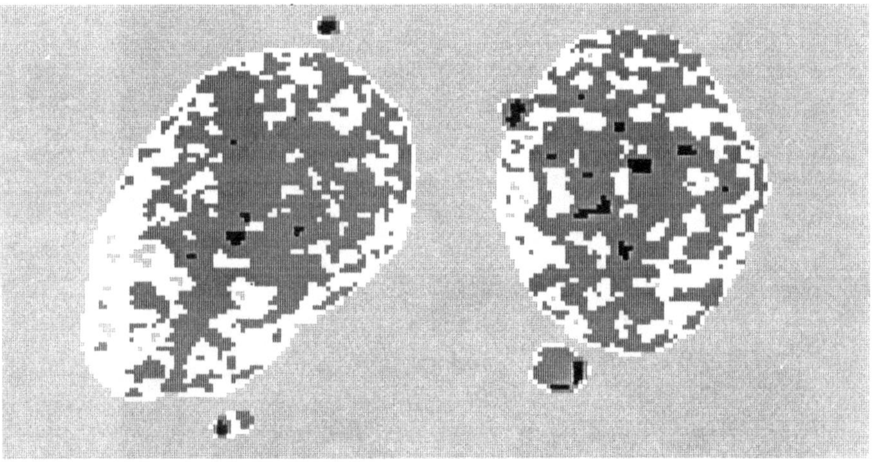

Fig. 11. Digital image of nuclei with micronuclei. DNA of CHO cells (treated with $6 \times 10^{-4} M$ MMS) was stained with Feulgen stain, and the images captured by the Cell Analyzer at 60+ magnification. The images were segmented into nuclear material and background. From the optical density measurements of the picture elements (*pixels*) in the nucleus, the amount of high, medium and low density chromatin was calculated, shown as *black*, *grey* and *white pixels*. The number, frequency, size, shape, amount of DNA, distribution of DNA and other texture parameters in the nuclei and micronuclei can be computed from such data. Scanning for nuclei and micronuclei and feature analysis can be performed in a fully automated manner

development in the Cancer Imaging Section of the B.C. Cancer Research Centre, incorporated into a device such as the Cell Analyzer (Palcic and Jaggi 1990; Jaggi et al. 1989). If used in a scanning mode, imaging the mathematical transformation of spectral information, stained DNA, nuclei and micronuclei can be readily detected and segmented from the cytoplasm. Figure 11 shows a picture of a nucleus and micronucleus imaged by a simulated system of a Solid State Microscope. Size, DNA amount, shape and texture features could also be determined while the slide is being scanned. When the Solid State Microscope is developed, its usefulness for the scoring of micronuclei in large-scale experiments will be validated.

References

Abe T, Isemura T, Kikuchi Y (1984) Micronuclei in human bone-marrow cells: evaluation of the micronucleus test using human leukemia patients treated with antileukemic agents. Mutat Res 130: 113–120

Blakey DH, Duncan AMV, Wargovich MJ, Goldberg MT, Bruce WR, Heddle JA (1985) Detection of nuclear anomalies in the colonic epithelium of the mouse. Cancer Res 45: 242–249

Bruce WR, Heddle JA (1979) The mutagenic activity of 61 different agents as determined by micronucleus, salmonella and sperm anomaly assays. Can J Genet Cytol 21: 319–334

Callisen HH, Pincu M, Norman A (1986) Feasibility of automating the micronucleus assay. Anal Quant Cytol Histol 8: 219–223

Cole RJ, Taylor N, Cole J, Arlett CF (1981) Short-term tests for transplacentally active carcinogens. I. Micronucleus formation in fetal and maternal mouse erythroblasts. Mutat Res 80: 141–157

Fenech M, Morley A (1985a) Solutions to the kinetic problem in the micronucleus assay. Cytobios 43: 233–246

Fenech M, Morley A (1985b) Measurement of micronuclei in lymphocytes. Mutat Res 147: 29–36

Fenech M, Morley A (1986) Cytokinesis-block micronucleus method in human lymphocytes: effect of in vivo ageing and low dose X-irradiation. Mutat Res 161: 193–198

Fontham E, Correa P, Rodriguez E, Lin Y (1986) Validation of smoking history with the micronuclei test. In: Hoffmann D, Harris CC (eds) Mechanisms in tobacco carcinogenesis. Cold Spring Harbor Laboratory, Cold Spring Harbor NY, pp 113–119 (Banbury report 23)

Henderson L, Cole R, Cole J, Cole H, Aghamohammadi Z, Regan T (1984) Sister-chromatid exchange and micronucleus induction as indicators of genetic damage in maternal and fetal cells. Mutat Res 126: 47–52

Högstedt B, Nilsson PG, Mitelman F (1981) Micronuclei in erythropoietic bone marrow cells: relation to cytogenetic pattern and prognosis in acute nonlymphocytic leukemia. Cancer Genet Cytogenet 3: 185–193

Högstedt B, Åkesson B, Axell K, Gullberg B, Mitelman F, Pero RW, Skerfving S, Welinder H (1983) Increased frequency of lymphocyte micronuclei in workers producing reinforced polyester resin with low exposure to styrene. Scand J Work Environ Health 49: 271–276

Jaggi B, Deen MJ, Palcic B (1989) Design of a Solid State Microscope. Opt Eng 28: 675–687

Jenssen D, Ramel C (1980) The micronucleus test as part of a short-term mutagenicity test program for the prediction of carcinogenicity evaluated by 143 agents tested. Mutat Res 75: 191–192

Lähdetie J (1986) Micronucleated spermatids in the seminal fluid of smokers and nonsmokers. Mutat Res 172: 255–263

MacGregor JT, Wehr CM, Langlois RG (1983) A simple fluorescent staining procedure for micronuclei and RNA in erythrocytes using Hoechst 33258 and pyronin Y. Mutat Res 120: 269–275

Mandard AM, Duigou F, Marnay J, Masson P, Qiu SL, Yi JS, Barrellier P, Lebigot G (1987) Analysis of the results of the micronucleus test in patients presenting upper digestive tract cancers and in non-cancerous subjects. Int J Cancer 39: 442–444

Meretoja T, Järventaus H, Sorsa M, Vainio H (1978) Chromosome aberrations in lymphocytes of workers exposed to styrene. Scand J Work Environ Health 4 [Suppl 2]: 259–264

Munoz N, Hayashi M, Lu JB, Wahrendorf J, Crespi M, Bosch FX (1987) Effect of riboflavin, retinol, and zinc on micronuclei of buccal mucosa and of esophagus: a randomized double-blind intervention study in China. JNCI 79: 687–691

Nordenson I, Beckman L (1984) Chromosomal aberrations in lymphocytes of workers exposed to low levels of styrene. Hum Hered 34: 178–182

Palcic B, Jaggi B (1990) Image cytometry system for morphometric measurements of live cells. In: Wise DL (ed) Bioinstrumentation: developments and applications. Butterworth, Stoneham MD (in press)

Parvez Z, Kormano M, Satokari K, Moncada R, Eklund R (1987) Induction of mitotic micronuclei by X-ray contrast media in human peripheral lymphocytes. Mutat Res 188: 233–239

Picker JD, Fox DP (1986) Do curried foods produce micronuclei in buccal epithelial cells? Mutat Res 171: 185–188

Raafat M, El-Gerzawi S, Stich HF (1984) Detection of mutagenicity in urothelial cells of bilharzial patients by "the micronucleus test". J Egypt Natl Cancer Inst 1: 63–73

Rabello-Gay MN, Carvalho MI, Otto PA, Targa HJ (1985) The effects of age, sex and diet on the clastogenic action of cyclophosphamide in mouse bone marrow. Mutat Res 158: 181–188

Reali D, DiMarino F, Bahramandpour S, Carducci A, Barale R, Loprieno N (1987) Micronuclei in exfoliated urothelial cells and urine mutagenicity in smokers. Mutat Res 192: 145–149

Ronen A, Heddle JA (1984) Site-specific induction of nuclear anomalies (apoptotic bodies and micronuclei) by carcinogens in mice. Cancer Res 44: 1536–1540

Rosin MP, German J (1985) Evidence for chromosome instability in vivo in Bloom syndrome: increased numbers of micronuclei in exfoliated cells. Hum Genet 71: 187–191

Rosin MP, Ochs HD (1986) In vivo chromosomal instability in ataxia-telangiectasia homozygotes and heterozygotes. Hum Genet 74: 335–340

Schlegel R, MacGregor JT (1984) The persistence of micronucleated erythrocytes in the peripheral circulation of normal and splenectomized Fischer 344 rats: implications for cytogenetic screening. Mutat Res 127: 169–174

Stich HF (1986a) The use of micronuclei in tracing the genotoxic damage in the oral mucosa of tobacco users. In: Hoffmann D, Harris CC (eds) Mechanisms in tobacco

carcinogenesis. Cold Spring Harbor Laboratory, Cold Spring Harbor NY, pp 99–111 (Banbury report 23)
Stich HF (1986b) Reducing the genotoxic damage in the oral mucosa of betel quid/tobacco chewers. In: Shankel DM et al. (eds) Antimutagenesis and anticarcinogenesis mechanisms. Plenum, New York, pp 381–391
Stich HF (1987) Micronucleated exfoliated cells as indicators for genotoxic damage and as markers in chemoprevention trials. J Nutr Growth Cancer 4: 9–18
Stich HF, Rosin MP (1983) Quantitating the synergistic effect of smoking and alcohol consumption with the micronucleus test on human buccal mucosa cells. Int J Cancer 31: 305–308
Stich HF, Rosin MP (1985) Towards a more comprehensive evaluation of a genotoxic hazard in man. Mutat Res 150: 43–50
Stich HF, Yohn DS (1970) Viruses and chromosomes. Prog Med Virol 12: 78–127
Stich HF, Curtis JR, Parida BB (1982a) Application of the micronucleus test to exfoliated cells of high cancer risk groups: tobacco chewers. Int J Cancer 30: 553–559
Stich HF, Stich W, Parida BB (1982b) Elevated frequency of micronucleated cells in the buccal mucosa of individuals at high risk for oral cancer: betel quid chewers. Cancer Lett 17: 125–134
Stich HF, Stich W, Rosin MP, Vallejera MO (1984) Use of the micronucleus test to monitor the effect of vitamin A, beta-carotene and canthaxanthin on the buccal mucosa of betel nut/tobacco chewers. Int J Cancer 34: 745–750
Stich HF, Hornby AP, Dunn BP (1985) A pilot beta-carotene intervention trial with Inuits using smokeless tobacco. Int J Cancer 36: 321–327
Stich HF, Rosin MP, Hornby AP, Mathew B, Sankaranarayanan R, Krishnan Nair M (1988) Remission of oral leukoplakias and micronuclei in tobacco/betel quid chewers treated with beta-carotene and with beta-carotene plus vitamin A. Int J Cancer 42: 195–199
Wargovich MJ, Goldberg MT, Newmark HL, Bruce WR (1983) Nuclear aberrations as a short-term test for genotoxicity to the colon: evaluation of nineteen agents in mice. JNCI 71: 133–137

*Identification of Occupational Cancer Risks Using a Population-Based Cancer Registry**

P.R. Band, J.J. Spinelli, R.P. Gallagher, W.J. Threlfall, V.T.Y. Ng, J. Moody, D. Raynor, L.M. Svirchev, D. Kan, and M. Wong**

Division of Epidemiology, Biometry and Occupational Oncology, Cancer Control Agency of British Columbia, 600 West 10th Avenue, Vancouver, B.C. V5Z 4E6, Canada

Introduction

Population-based cancer registries provide a unique opportunity for epidemiologic research aimed at identifying occupational cancer risks. However, this potential has been underutilized due to insufficient information on occupation and industry or data on important confounders such as cigarette smoking, alcohol consumption and socio-economic status (McCrea Curnen et al. 1984). Due to these limitations, occupational studies using population-based cancer registries for case ascertainment have generally focussed on studies of occupational risks associated with a single tumor site (Jarvisalo et al. 1984; McLaughlin et al. 1987; Pearce et al. 1986a,b), and have rarely encompassed the broad spectrum of human malignancies with the possibility to control for confounding variables (Williams et al. 1977).

We have undertaken a study to determine occupational cancer risk in male cancer patients in British Columbia (B.C.), the most westerly province of Canada with a population of 2.7 million. Cancer care and services in this province are under the responsibility of the Cancer Control Agency of British Columbia (CCABC), which operates two cancer centres as well as the population-based British Columbia Cancer Registry (BCCR). In this report, the study methodology and preliminary data on occupational risk in non-Hodgkin's lymphoma and squamous cell lung cancer will be presented.

Methods and Procedures

The British Columbia Cancer Registry

In British Columbia, cancer has been a notifiable disease since 1932, although good ascertainment was not achieved until 1969. Since 1969, duplicates of all

* Supported by grant # 6610–1395–53 from NHRDP, Health and Welfare Canada, and by grants from the Workers' Compensation Board of British Columbia and the Vancouver Foundation.

** The authors are indebted to Mrs. Jean van den Broek for secretarial assistance.

bustion products have been associated with scrotal tumors in chimney sweeps since as early as 1775 (Pott 1775). The carbonization of bituminous coal to produce coke also emits complex organic mixtures similar to coal combustion emissions. Epidemiological studies (Lloyd 1971; Redmond et al. 1972, 1976, 1979) revealed that coke oven workers were at an increased risk of mortality from lung cancer, prostate cancer, and kidney cancer. Mazumdar et al. (1975) showed a dose-response relationship between exposure of coke oven emissions and development of lung cancer in coke oven workers.

A China national cancer survey for the cancer mortality rate during 1973–1975 first revealed that Xuan Wei County in rural Southern China has an unusually high lung cancer mortality rate (Li et al. 1979). A subsequent clinical survey conducted at a local hospital confirmed this finding (Coordinative Group of Lung Cancer in Xiang Wei District 1979). These survey results caused great public health concern and prompted investigations into lung cancer problems in Xuan Wei. In this report, we use the Xuan Wei lung cancer study as a case study to evaluate lung cancer risks from exposure to the complex organic mixtures of coal and wood combustion emissions.

Xuan Wei Background

Xuan Wei county, which encompasses a total area of 6257 km^2, is located in northeastern Yunnan Province, China. The county is situated on a plateau with high mountains, its altitude ranging from 920 m to 2866 m. The county has a population of 1 million people, who live in 20 communes. Ninety percent or more are farmers. Most residents (94%) are Han, the predominant ethnic group in China. Local industries include coal mining; production of fertilizer, solvent, and cement; and electric power generation. All these plants were built after 1960. More than 40% of Xuan Wei males smoke tobacco, and less than 1% of Xuan Wei females smoke. The tobacco products used are commercial cigarettes and locally grown tobaccos. Tobacco is often smoked through water pipes (He et al. 1986).

High concentrations of air pollutants are generated in Xuan Wei homes (Mumford et al. 1987). In Xuan Wei, home heating is required in the winter months. For generations, Xuan Wei residents have used one of three fuels, "smoky" coal, "smokeless" coal, or wood, for domestic heating and cooking. Smoky coal is equivalent to medium-volatile bituminous coal with 0.2% sulfur, 20% ash, and a heating value of 27.1 MJ/kg (Mumford et al. 1987). Burning of smoky coal generates high concentrations of smoke in the homes. Smokeless coal is a low-grade coal with 1.9% sulfur, 49% ash, and a heating value of 14.5 MJ/kg. Before it is burned, the pulverized smokeless coal is usually mixed with clay to form briquets. A much lower level of smoke is generated by smokeless coal than by smoky coal. Both types of coal come from small local mines distributed throughout the county (see Fig. 1). Women usually are responsible for most household chores, which include starting the fire and

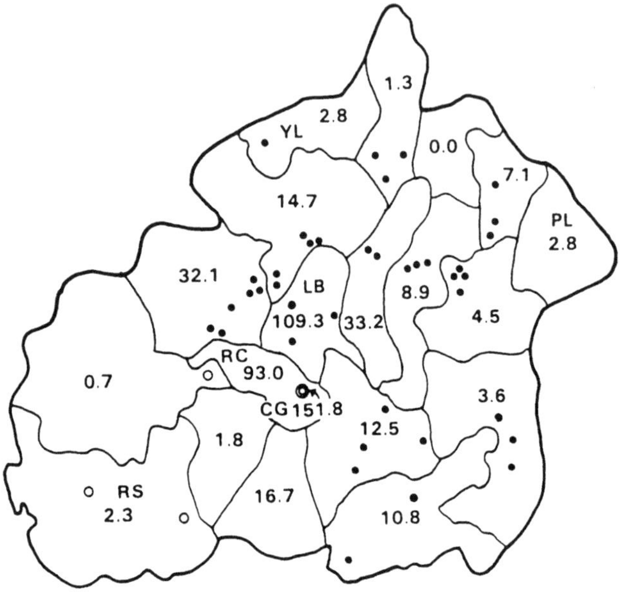

Fig. 1. Map of Xuan Wei County, showing commune boundaries, each commune's unadjusted annual lung cancer mortality rate per 100000 (both sexes, 1973–75), and mines supplying domestic coal: • smoky coal; o smokeless coal. Designated communes: high mortality – *CG*, Cheng Guan; *LB*, Lai Bin; *RC*, Rong Cheng; low mortality – *PL*, Pu Li, *RS*, Re Shui; *YL*, Yang Liu. (From Mumford et al. 1987, with permission; copyright 1987 by the AAAS)

cooking. A survey of 64 Xuan Wei residents showed that women on average spend about 7 h near the household fire, and men spend 3.7 h near the fire. Men spend more time (9.6 h) working outdoors than women (6.7 h; He et al. 1986).

Characteristics of Lung Cancer in Xuan Wei

High Lung Cancer Mortality Rate

In Xuan Wei, respiratory disease is the number one leading cause of death (He et al. 1986). Of the Xuan Wei deaths due to cancer, the mortality rate for lung cancer is the highest, followed distantly by those for liver cancer and stomach cancer. In the overall statistics for China, stomach cancer is the leading cause of cancer deaths. Lung cancer in Xuan Wei is the only cancer for which the mortality exceeds China's national average (Li et al. 1979). Lung cancer reported in this paper includes carcinomas of the lung parenchyma, bronchus, and trachea. Table 1 presents the annual lung cancer mortality rates in Xuan Wei. The lung cancer mortality rate for women in Xuan Wei is the highest in

Table 1. Annual lung cancer mortality rates in China and the United States. (From Mumford et al. 1987, with permission; copyright 1987 by the AAAS)

	Mortality rate (per 100000)						
	Unadjusted			Age-adjusted to 1964 China population		Age-adjusted to 1970 US population	
	Males	Females	Combined	Males	Females	Males	Females
China, 1973–75			5.0	6.8	3.2	12.3	5.7
United States, 1970	53.7	12.0		30.0	6.3	53.7	12.0
Yunnan Province, 1973–75			2.8	4.3	1.5	6.9	2.5
Xuan Wei County, 1973–79	27.0	24.5		27.7	25.3	43.2	38.7
Three high-mortality Xuan Wei communes (Cheng Guan, Lai Bin, Rong Cheng), 1973–79	114.4	120.6		118.0	125.6	186.8	193.4

China, and the rate for Xuan Wei men is among China's highest (Department of Public Health, People's Republic of China 1979).

Lung Cancer Types

A clinical study conducted in a high-mortality commune, Lai Bin, showed that of 115 sputum specimens from lung cancer patients, 58% contained cells with squamous carcinomas, and 28% contained cells with adenocarcinomas; cells in the remaining 14% of the specimens were characterized by mixed-cell, undifferentiated, or alveolar carcinomas (Coordinative Group of Lung Cancer in Xiang Wei 1979). In general, percent distribution of these cancer types is similar in males and females, even though females have a slightly higher percentage of the adenocarcinoma cell type (31%) than males (25%) and a lower percentage of the squamous carcinoma cell type (55%) than males (62%).

Similarity of Lung Cancer Rates in Males and Females

In most countries, the lung cancer mortality rates for males are higher than those for females. This difference is mainly due to more cigarette smoking and higher occupational exposure in males than in females. In China overall, the ratio of male-to-female lung cancer mortality is 2.1 (Li et al. 1979). In contrast, the corresponding ratio in Xuan Wei is only 1.09. In Lai Bin, one of the communes with a high rate of lung cancer, the ratio is 0.87, indicating that the lung cancer mortality rate for females is higher than that for males. The lung cancer mortality rates for age groups of 45–49, 50–54, and 55–59 years are higher in females (407.8, 669.9, and 904.0 per 100000, respectively) than in males (348.5, 513.7, and 849.4 per 100000, respectively) in the three communes with high mortality rates for lung cancer (He et al. 1986). These findings suggest that domestic factors are most likely associated with lung cancer in Xuan Wei females.

Lung Cancer Death at an Early Age

The Xuan Wei data plotted in Figs. 2 and 3 show that, for both males and females, the 55- to 59-year age group has the highest mortality rate for lung cancer, in contrast to the age-specific data for China as a whole, for which the age group of 70–74 has the highest lung cancer mortality rate. The average age at death of lung cancer patients in Xuan Wei (54.2 for males and 53.7 for females) is 6 years lower than that of the China national average (He et al. 1986). In comparison with other areas in China with high lung cancer rates, the age at death is also the lowest in Xuan Wei. These findings suggest that (a) Xuan Wei residents are exposed to the cancer-causing agent at an early age and thus the disease is manifest at an early age, and/or (b) the cancer-causing agent is very potent and is latent for only a short period before manifestation of the disease.

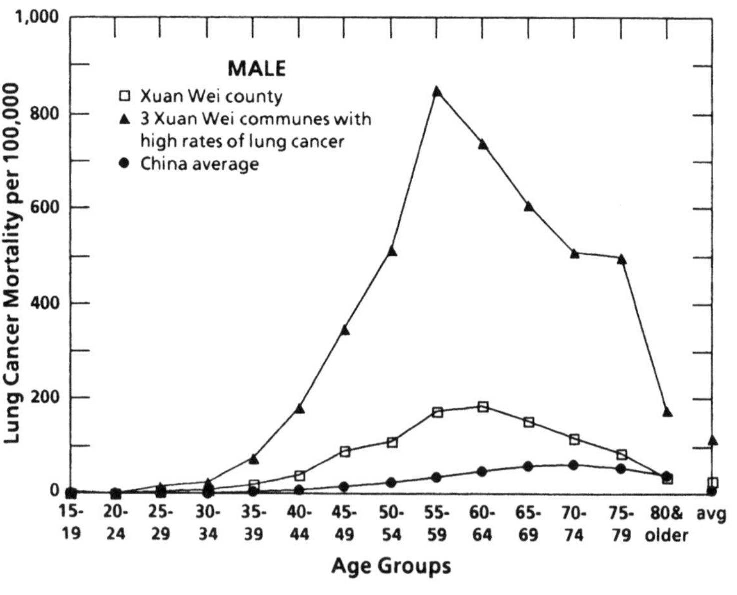

Fig. 2. Age-specific lung cancer mortality rate for Xuan Wei (1973–79) and China (1973–1975), male population

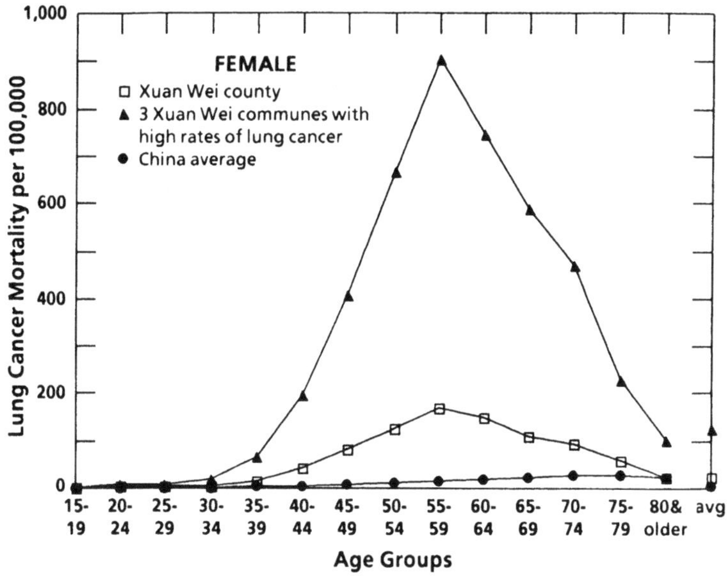

Fig. 3. Age-specific lung cancer mortality rate for Xuan Wei (1973–79) and China (1973–1975), female population

Geographical Variation in Lung Cancer Mortality Rates in Xuan Wei

There is a wide variation among Xuan Wei communes in lung cancer mortality rates, ranging from 0 to 151.8/100000, as shown in Fig. 1. The central communes, Cheng Guan, Lai Bin, and Rong Cheng have the highest rates. Most communes located in the peripheral regions showed lower mortality rates for lung cancer. This suggests that the specific environmental determinants of lung cancer may be geographically related.

Xuan Wei Lung Cancer and Contributing Factors of Occupation and Tobacco Smoke

Studies have shown that the causes of lung cancer are mostly environmental (Dean 1962; Coy et al. 1968; Mazumdar et al. 1975). The relevant environmental factors contributing to lung cancer are tobacco smoke, occupation, and residence-related air pollution. Tobacco smoke is known for causing lung cancer in man (International Agency for Research on Cancer 1986). Thus, it is essential to investigate the role of tobacco smoking in lung cancer mortality in Xuan Wei. In Xuan Wei, even though the smoking rate for females (0.2%) is much lower than the male rate (42.7%), the lung cancer mortality rates for

Table 2. Comparison of two Xuan Wei communes for lung-cancer mortality, cigarette smoking, and domestic fuel use. (From Chapman et al. 1988)

Commune	Lung cancer mortality rate[a] (per 100000)	With history of cigarette smoking (%)		Population using smoky coal (%)
		Male	Female	
Lai Bin	109.3	44.0	0.05	89.7
Re Shui	2.3	49.1	0.07	0[b]

[a] Unadjusted annual lung cancer mortality, 1973–1975.
[b] 66.6% of Re Shui residents use wood, and 33.4% of these residents use smokeless coal.

females and males are similar (25.3/100000 for females and 27.7/100000 for males).

The results of a 1982 survey of tobacco smoking in two Xuan Wei communes, one with a high lung cancer rate and one with a low rate, also suggested that smoking is not the main factor contributing to the high lung cancer mortality in Xuan Wei (He et al. 1986). As shown in Table 2, the commune with the high lung cancer rate, Lai Bin, and the low lung cancer commune, Re Shui, have similar smoking rates, but the lung cancer mortality rates are very different. These observations suggest that factors other than tobacco smoking contribute to the high lung mortality rate for cancer in Xuan Wei.

A clinical survey was conducted in Xuan Wei in the late 1970s. In a population of 91187 people surveyed, 262 lung cancer cases (287/100000) were detected. According to occupation, the detection rate in farmers, office workers, and coal miners was 339, 118, and 15 per 100000, respectively (Coordinative Group of Lung Cancer in Xiang Wei District 1979). This finding suggests that Xuan Wei lung cancer is not associated with nonagricultural occupations.

Lung Cancer and Indoor Air Pollution from Coal and Wood Combustion in Xuan Wei

The above observations suggested that the high mortality rate from lung cancer in Xuan Wei can not be attributed to tobacco smoke or occupational exposure. Because Xuan Wei residents, especially women, have been exposed to high concentrations of coal and wood combustion indoors and because incomplete combustion products are a rich source of carcinogens, the relationship between domestic fuel use and Xuan Wei lung cancer was investigated. A 1982 fuel survey (He et al. 1986) conducted in 11 Xuan Wei communes showed that the

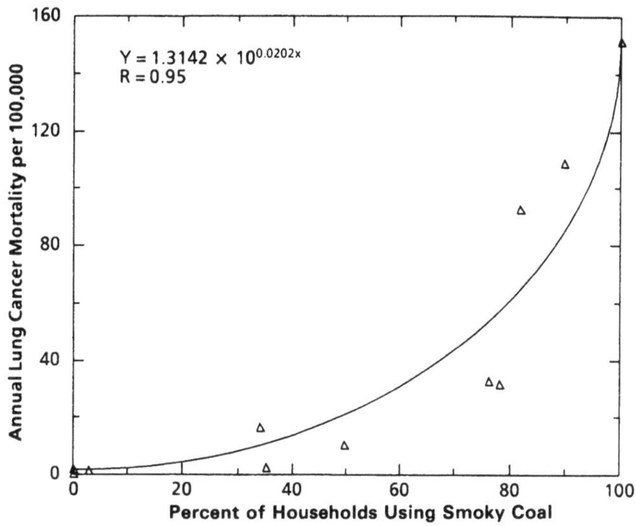

Fig. 4. Percentage of households using smoky coal before 1958, and 1973–75 unadjusted annual lung cancer mortality in 11 Xuan Wei communes

logarithm of the lung cancer mortality rate was highly correlated ($R=0.95$) with the percentage of households using smoky coal before 1958 (Fig. 4). No correlation was found between lung cancer and percentage of households using wood. This finding generated the hypothesis that indoor air pollution from domestic use of smoky coal is the prime determinant of lung cancer in Xuan Wei. Under a China-US agreement (China-US Protocol 1980), we are conducting interdisciplinary studies to examine the relationship between Xuan Wei lung cancer and indoor exposure of coal and wood combustion emissions in Xuan Wei. The up-to-date results are presented below.

Indoor Air Monitoring, Characterization, and Toxicological Studies

Indoor air and outdoor air were sampled in a central commune, Cheng Guan, where mortality was Xuan Wei's highest (151.8/100 000) and smoky coal is the major fuel, and in a southwestern commune, Re Shui, where mortality is low (2.3/100 000) and wood (67%) and smokeless coal (33%) are the fuels used. Inhalable particles ($<10\,\mu$m, or PM_{10}) and semivolatile organic compounds were collected by filters and XAD-2 resin from four homes of each commune during cooking periods (Mumford et al. 1987). The particles were examined by electron microscope to determine size. The percentage of organic mass extractable by dichloromethane in the particles was determined. Polycyclic aromatic hydrocarbons were analyzed by gas chromatography and mass spectrometry

(Nishioka et al. 1982). The organic extracts were also fractionated into compound classes to identify the biologically active compounds (Petersen and Chuang 1982). The Ames *Salmonella*/microsome mutation assay (Ames et al. 1975), which has been widely used to screen environmental agents for potential carcinogenicity, was used to determine the mutagenicity of the organic extracts and fractions. The organic extracts of particles emitted from indoor combustion were also bioassayed in the L5178Y $TK^{+/-}$ mouse lymphoma cell mutation assay to confirm the mutagenicity of these organic emissions in a mammalian cell system. The method of Clive et al. (1979) was used for the lymphoma assay. A skin tumor initiation assay was also conducted to assess the tumorigenicity of the emission samples (Mumford et al. in press). Female Sencar mice were initiated topically with organic extracts of the indoor combustion emission particles; mice were dosed at 1, 2, 5, 10, and 20 mg/mouse at week 1 and then promoted with the tumor promoter 12-*O*-tetradecanoylphorbol-13-acetate (TPA) twice weekly for the subsequent 26 weeks. Data reported here are the results of scoring papillomas after 26 weeks of promotion.

Peak Exposure, Particle Size, and Chemical Analysis of Emissions

As shown in Table 3, the indoor concentrations of PM_{10} during combustion of smoky coal and wood were very high (24.4 mg/m^3 and 22.3 mg/m^3, respect-

Table 3. Characteristics of indoor air particles in Xuan Wei homes during cooking[a]

	Smoky coal[a]	Wood	Smokeless coal
Particulate concentration (mg/m^3)	24.4 ± 3.3	22.3 ± 2.0[a]	1.8
Particle size (percent of submicron particles)	51	6	N.A.
Organic mass extractable (percent)	72.3 ± 6.7	55.1 ± 7.0	27.0
PAH concentrations[b] (μg/m^3)			
Benzo[*a*]anthracene	25.1 ± 5.0	4.0 ± 1.1	1.0
5-Methylchrysene	7.3 ± 2.7	0.2 ± 0.06	0.2
Benzofluoranthene	22.7 ± 4.6	2.7 ± 0.7	1.9
Benzo[*a*]pyrene	14.7 ± 3.0	3.1 ± 1.0	0.6
Indeno[1,2,3-*cd*]pyrene	8.4 ± 3.9	2.0 ± 0.6	0.5
Dibenzo[*ae*]pyrene	11.7 ± 4.2	0.2 ± 0.07	0.6
Dibenz[*aj*]acridene	0.7	BDL	0.007

[a] Data from four homes (mean ± SEM) except data on smokeless coal, particle size, and dibenz[*aj*]acridene are from one home.

[b] Compounds presented are the ones that showed sufficient evidence of carcinogenicity in experimental animals (International Agency for Research on Cancer 1983).

BDL, below detection limit; N.A., data not available.

ively). These concentrations are more than 100 times the US 24-h ambient air standard for PM_{10} (*Federal Register* 1984). The indoor particulate concentrations during combustion of smokeless coal were much lower. The outdoor concentrations, 0.58 mg/m^3 and 0.05 mg/m^3 for the Cheng Guan and the Re Shui communes, respectively, were much lower than the indoor concentrations.

Electron microscopy studies showed that 51% of the particles from smoky coal combustion were less than 1 μm in diameter, and most particles were spherical (Mumford et al. 1987). In contrast to smoky coal emission particles, only 6% of wood particles were smaller than 1 μm. Many large, unburned fuel particles were found in the wood combustion emission. Organic extraction studies showed that more than 70% of the particles emitted from smoky coal combustion were organic-extractable, in contrast to the wood and the smokeless coal emission particles, which had organic-extractable mass fractions of only 55% and 27%, respectively (Table 3). Much lower content of organic-extractable matter was found in the outdoor air particles of the Cheng Guan (42%) and Re Shui (13.3%) communes.

Fractionation of the organic extract of the smoky coal emission particles showed it contained 36.4% aromatic compounds, 35% of moderately polar compounds, and 30.8% polar compounds; whereas the organic extract of wood combustion particles contained mostly polar compounds (78.3%), and only 7.7% of the mass was found in the aromatic fraction (Table 4). A mutagenicity study of the fractions showed that the aromatic and the polar fractions of the smoky coal organic extract exhibited the highest mutagenic activity (Mumford et al. 1987). A recent study of mouse skin tumor initiation showed that the aromatic fraction exhibited the highest activity. (X. Li et al., unpublished data). Quantitative gas chromatography and mass spectrometry analysis showed that, in comparison with wood combustion emissions, the organic extract of smoky coal combustion particles contained higher concentrations of the carcinogenic PAH, methylated PAH, and nitrogen-containing heterocyclic compounds (Table 3). The polar fraction of the smoky coal sample included nitrogen-containing compounds (e.g., diphenyl pyrrole, acridine, and methyl acridinone) and also some oxygen-containing compounds (e.g., fatty acids, fatty acid esters, aromatic ketones, and quinones). Low levels of these organic compounds were found in the smokeless coal emission (Mumford et al. 1987).

Mutagenicity and Tumorigenicity of the Organic Extracts from Combustion Emission Particles

The mutagenicity studies in bacterial and mammalian cell assays showed that the organic extracts of all three types of combustion emission particles induced mutation. All the XAD samples showed little mutagenic activity in the Ames assay (Mumford et al. 1987). The organic extracts of the emission particles also showed tumor initiation activity in the mouse skin assay (Table 5). In all three assays, the smoky coal samples consistently showed much higher biological

Table 4. Fractionation and mutagenicity of organic extracts from combustion emission particles (PM_{10}) collected in Xuan Wei homes during cooking

Fraction	Smoky coal		Wood		Smokeless coal	
	Mass (mg/m^3)	Mutagenicity[a] ($\times 10^3$ rev/m^3)	Mass (mg/m^3)	Mutagenicity ($\times 10^3$ rev/m^3)	Mass (mg/m^3)	Mutagenicity ($\times 10^3$ rev/m^3)
Neat sample	22.7	58.9	15.9	11.1	0.5	1.3
Aliphatic compounds (hexane)	1.1	0	0.2	0	0.02	0
Aromatic compounds (hexane/benzene)	8.2	18.1	1.2	3.1	0.2	0.5
Moderately polar compounds (dichloromethane)	7.9	8.7	2.3	4.4	0.1	0.3
Polar compounds (methanol)	7.0	24.4	12.4	5.0	0.2	0.4

[a] Mutagenicity was determined in *Salmonella typhimurium* TA98 with S9. Each sample was solvent exchanged to dimethyl sulfoxide and tested at a minimum of five doses in triplicate. The slope of the initial linear portion ($R^2 \geq 0.90$) of each dose-response curve was calculated by least squares linear regression. Data represent one home in each commune.
rev/m^3, revertants per cubic meter of air.

Table 5. Comparative potency of organic extracts from combustion emission particles (PM_{10}) collected in Xuan Wei homes during cooking

Fuel type	Salmonella mutagenicity TA98 (+S9)		Mouse lymphoma mutagenicity (+S9)		Mouse skin tumor initiation		Human lung cancer mortality per 100 000
	Revertants per m^3 [a]	Ratio to wood	Mutation frequency per m^3 [a]	Ratio to wood	Papillomas per m^3	Ratio to wood	
Smoky coal	58.9	5.3	1406.5	4.8	13.8	6.6	151.8
Wood	11.1	1.0	292.6	1.0	2.1	1.0	2.3[b]
Smokeless coal	1.3	0.12	42.5	0.15	0.2	0.1	

[a] Each sample was tested at a minimum of five doses. The rat liver homogenate of the S9 fraction was added for metabolic activation in the two mutagenesis assays. A sample was considered positive if a dose-response relation was observed. The slope of the initial linear portion of each dose-response curve was calculated by least-squares linear regression ($R^2 \geq 0.85$) to obtain the potency per microgram of organic extract. The potency per cubic meter of air for each type of emission was calculated by multiplying the potency per microgram of organic extract by the micrograms of organic extract per cubic meter of air. Data presented are from a representive home in each commune.

[b] Lung cancer mortality rate in Re Shui, where 67% of the residents used wood and 33% used smokeless coal.

activity than the wood or the smokeless coal samples. Good concordance among the three assays was observed. A complete carcinogenesis assay in Sencar mouse skin also showed that the smoky coal extract induces squamous cell carcinomas as a complete carcinogen when applied dermally twice weekly for 52 weeks at 2 mg per mouse per week without TPA promotion (Mumford et al. in press). The results of these short-term genetic and carcinogenic assays are in agreement with human lung cancer data, showing that smoky coal emissions are more potent than wood or smokeless coal emissions.

Epidemiological Case-Control Study

A case-control study is currently ongoing in Xuan Wei. The control subjects, who are matched with lung cancer patients by age ($\pm$ 4 years) and sex, are randomly selected throughout the county. Table 6 shows the preliminary findings from the first 33 case-control pairs of males and 39 pairs of females (Chapman et al. 1988). The results show that the risk of lung cancer in Xuan Wei is associated with the use of smoky coal. In general, a higher odds ratio was found in females than in males. This may be attributed to the longer time that females spend near the fire every day. Also, a general trend indicated the odds ratio increased with the duration of using smoky coal.

Summary

The study of Xuan Wei fuel use and lung cancer mortality and also the interim case-control study suggested an association between domestic smoky coal use and Xuan Wei lung cancer. The collaborative studies of physical characterization, chemical analysis, and toxicology further substantiated this linkage. The Xuan Wei residents who used smoky coal inhaled extremely high concentrations of mostly submicron-sized particles, which can be inhaled and deposited effectively deep in the lung. These fine particles were composed mostly of organic compounds (72%), including mutagenic and carcinogenic organic

Table 6. Interim odds ratios associated with smoky coal use in Xuan Wei lung cancer cases and controls. (From Chapman et al., 1988)

Time using smoky coal	Males (33 pairs)	Females (39 pairs)
Now	1.5	2.6
20 years ago	1.3	2.9
At age 12	4.0	3.7

compounds, especially in the aromatic and polar fractions. These residents were exposed to polycyclic aromatic compounds, such as benzo[*a*]pyrene, at comparable or higher levels than those measured in coke oven plants and other occupational environments (International Agency for Research on Cancer 1984). In comparison with wood and smokeless coal combustion emissions, the organic extracts of smoky coal emission particles showed much higher activity of genotoxicity and carcinogenicity. These results all point to a strong etiological link between the complex organic mixtures from smoky coal emissions and Xuan Wei lung cancer.

This study and studies reported by other investigators (de Koning et al. 1984) suggested little association between indoor open-fire wood smoke and lung cancer. The less efficient lung deposition of the larger particles from wood combustion, as well as the lower concentrations of biologically active organic compounds, may contribute to the low rate of lung cancer in the wood-burning communes. As to the smokeless coal emissions, the lower particulate concentration and the lower organic content of the particles emitted may also contribute to the low lung cancer rate in the commune using this fuel.

In conclusion, the complex organic mixtures from combustion emissions are genotoxic and carcinogenic in animal and in vitro assays. The magnitude of the cancer risks from the complex organic mixtures in man depends on the degree of the exposure, the types of the compounds contained in the mixtures, and the concentrations of these biologically active compounds present in the combustion emissions.

Acknowledgements. The authors wish to thank the investigators of the Institute of Environmental Health and Engineering in Beijing and the staff from the antiepidemic stations in Yunnan Province, Qu Jing Region, and Xuan Wei County for their assistance in field sampling and data collection. The authors also thank D. Bruce Harris of the US Environmental Protection Agency for his technical assistance in sampling. The research described in this article has been reviewed by the Health Effects Research Laboratory, US Environmental Protection Agency, and approved for publication. Approval does not signify that the contents necessarily reflect the views and policies of the Agency, nor does mention of trade names or commercial products constitute endorsement or recommendation for use.

References

Ames BW, McCann JM, Yamasaki E (1975) Methods for detecting carcinogens and mutagens with the *Salmonella*/mammalian microsome mutagenicity test. Mutat Res 31: 347–364

Chapman RS, He XZ, Jiang WZ, Yang R, Mumford JL, Harris DB (1988) The epidemiology of lung cancer in Xuan Wei, China: current progress, issues, and research strategies. Arch Environ Health 43: 180–185

China-US Protocol (1980) The China-U.S. Protocol, Annex 1, II.A. for scientific and technical cooperation in the field of environmental protection
Claxton LD, Huisingh JL (1980) Comparative mutagenic activity of organics from combustion sources. In: Sanders CL, Cross FT, Dagle GE, Mahaffey JA (eds) Pulmonary toxicology of respirable particles. CONF-791002 Department of Energy, US Government Printing Office, Washington pp 453–465 (DOE symposium ser 53)
Clive D, Johnson KO, Spector JFS, Batson AG, Brown MMM (1979) Validation and characterization of the L5178Y $TK^{+/-}$ mouse lymphoma mutagen assay system. Mutat Res 59: 61–108
Coordinative Group of Lung Cancer in Xiang Wei District (1979) Lung cancer in Xiang Wei District. Yunnan Med J 1979: 16–17
Coy P, Grzybowski S, Rower JF (1968) Lung cancer mortality according to birthplace. Can Med Assoc J 99: 476–483
Dean G (1962) Lung cancer in Australia. Med J Aust 1: 1003–1006
de Koning HW, Smith KR, Last JM (1984) Biomass fuel combustion and health. World Health Organization, Geneva (WHO EFP/84.64.)
Department of Public Health, the People's Republic of China (1979) Investigation and research of Chinese cancer mortality rates, chap 7. People's Public Health, Beijing, pp 148–174
Doll R, Peto R (1978) Cigarette smoking and bronchial carcinoma: dose and time relationship among regular smokers and lifelong non-smokers. J Epidemiol Community Health 32: 303–313
Federal Register (20 March 1984) p 10 416
He XZ, Cao SR, Jiang WZ, Yang RD, Xu CW (1986) Research on etiology of lung cancer in Xuan Wei. Institute of Environmental Health and Engineering, Chinese Academy of Preventive Medicine, Beijing
International Agency for Research on Cancer (IARC) (1983) IARC monographs on the evaluation of the carcinogenic risk of chemicals to humans, vol 32, pt 1. IARC, Lyon, pp 95–447
International Agency for Research on Cancer (IARC) (1984) Polycyclic aromatic compounds, industrial exposures in aluminum production, coal gasification, coke production and iron and steel founding. IARC, Lyon, pp 107–108. (IARC monogr on the evaluation of the carcinogenic risk of chemicals to humans, vol 34, pt 3)
International Agency for Research on Cancer (IARC) (1986) Tobacco smoking. IARC, Lyon (IARC monogr on the evaluation of carcinogenic risk of chemicals to humans, vol 38)
Ishinishi N, Koizumi A, McClellan RO, Stober W (eds) (1986) Carcinogenic and mutagenic effects of diesel engine exhaust. Elsevier, Amsterdam
Kamens RM, Rives GD, Perry JM, Bell DA, Paylor RF Jr, Claxton LD (1984) Mutagenic changes in dilute wood smoke as it ages and reacts with ozone and nitrogen dioxide: an outdoor chamber study. Environ Sci Technol 18: 523–530
Kinouchi T, Nishifuji K, Tsutsui H, Hoare SL, Ohnishi Y (1988) Mutagenicity and nitropyrene concentration of indoor air particulates exhausted from a kerosene heater. Jpn J Cancer Res (Gann) 79: 32–41
Lewtas J (1983) Evaluation of the mutagenicity and carcinogenicity of motor vehicle emissions in short-term bioassays. Environ Health Perspect 47: 141–152
Lewtas J (1985) Combustion emissions: characterization and comparison of their mutagenic and carcinogenic activity. In: Stich HF (ed) The workplace. CRC, Boca Raton Fl, pp 59–74 (Carcinogens and mutagens in the environment, vol 5)

Li JY et al. (eds) (1979) Atlas of cancer mortality in the People's Republic of China. China Map, Shanghai
Lloyd JW (1971) Long-term mortality study of steelworkers. V. Respiratory cancer in coke plant workers. J Occup Med 13(2): 53–68
Mazumdar S, Redmond C, Sollecito W, Sussman N (1975) An epidemiological study of exposure to coal tar pitch volatiles among coke oven workers. J Air Pollut Control Assoc 25(4): 382–389
Mumford JL, Lewtas J (1982) Mutagenicity and cytotoxicity of coal fly ash from fluidized-bed and conventional combustion. J Toxicol Environ Health 10: 565–586
Mumford JL, He XZ, Chapman RS, Cao SR, Harris DB, Li XM, Xian YL, Jiang WZ, Xu CW, Chuang JC, Wilson WE, Cooke M (1987) Lung cancer and indoor air pollution in Xuan Wei, China. Science 235: 217–220
Mumford JL, Helmes CT, Lee X, Seidenberg J, Nesnow S. Mouse skin tumorigenicity studies of indoor coal and wood combustion from homes of residents in Xuan Wei, China with high lung cancer mortality. Carcinogenesis (in press)
Nesnow S, Triplett L, Slaga TJ (1982) Comparative tumor-initiating activity of complex mixtures from environmental particulate emissions on SENCAR mouse skin. JNCI 68: 829–834
Nishioka MG, Petersen BA, Lewtas J (1982) Comparison of nitro-aromatic content and direct-acting mutagenicity of diesel emissions. In: Cooke M, Dennis AJ, Fisher GL (eds) Polynuclear aromatic hydrocarbons: physical and biological chemistry. Battelle, Columbus Oh, pp 603–613
Petersen BA, Chuang JC (1982) Methodology of fractionation and partition of diesel exhaust particulate samples. In: Lewtas J (ed) Toxicological effects of emissions from diesel engines. Elsevier, New York, pp 51–57
Pott P (1775) Cancer Scroti. In: The chirurgical works of Percival Pott. Printed by L Hawes, W Clarke, and R Collins, London pp 734–736
Redmond CK, Ciocco A, Lloyd JW, Rush HW (1972) Long term mortality study of steelworkers. VI. Mortality from malignant neoplasms among coke oven workers. J Occup Med 14: 621–629
Redmond CK, Strobino BR, Cypress RH (1976) Cancer experience among coke by-product workers. Ann NY Acad Sci 271: 102–115
Redmond C, Wieand HS, Rockette HE, Sass R, Weinberg G (1979) Long-term mortality experience of steelworkers. Report prepared by the University of Pittsburgh Graduate School of Public Health, Pittsburgh Pa (contract no HSM-99-71-32) for the National Institute of Occupational Safety and Health, Division of Surveillance, Hazard Evaluation, and Field Studies, Cincinnati
US Department of Health and Human Services (1982) The health consequences of smoking: a report of the Surgeon General. US Public Health Service, Washington, pp 13–196

Cancer Risks Due to Asbestos and Man-Made Fibres

J.C. McDonald

National Heart and Lung Institute, Brompton Hospital, Fulham Road, London SW3 6HP, United Kingdom

Introduction

Almost exactly 100 years ago, the mining and milling of asbestos began, reaching peak production in the early 1970s. Since then, because of the cancer hazard, the asbestos industry has gone into rapid decline and its very survival put in doubt. Production of manmade mineral fibres (MMMF) has followed a parallel trend, with a lag of about 50 years, and is now faced by similar fears. Few if any environmental agents have been subjected to such intense biological research as mineral fibres, for good reason, and their economic importance is equalled only by the threat they pose.

This paper will summarize what is reasonably well established on the epidemiology of asbestos-related malignant disease and then examine in more detail some results of recent research, including that on MMMF. Lung cancer and malignant mesothelioma are the main concern; cancers of the gastrointestinal tract, larynx and certain other sites have also been linked to asbestos exposure, but their total impact is relatively small and the nature of the association less clear. In a recent view, Doll and Peto (1987) concluded that, except for laryngeal cancer, there were insufficient grounds for attributing any of these diseases to asbestos. After an extensive examination of the epidemiological evidence on laryngeal cancer, Liddell (1988) remained unconvinced even for these tumours. Without more data these questions cannot be resolved.

For lung cancer and mesothelioma the situation is quite different. Although important differences in risk have been demonstrated with fibre type and industrial process, the overall impact of asbestos exposure on health is substantial. An indication of its magnitude is shown in Table 1 which summarizes the results of all cohort studies published to date. Even in the absence of information on age, sex, smoking and exposure intensity the consistent pattern of mortality is striking. The experience of cohorts exposed to the amphiboles and chrysotile-amphibole mixtures is closely similar but several times worse than those exposed to chrysotile only. This large difference is partly explained by the rarity of mesothelioma in the chrysotile-only cohorts but also be lesser risks from lung cancer and pneumoconiosis.

Recent Results in Cancer Research, Vol. 120

Table 1. Excess mortality in cohorts exposed to asbestos (%)

	Chrysotile only	Amphiboles only	Chrysotile-amphibole mixtures
Pneumoconiosis ($n=21$; male only)	83/4996 1.7%	102/2008 5.1%	254/6471 3.9%
Lung cancer ($n=42$)	02/5827 1.8%	137/2187 6.3%	772/10882 7.1%
Mesothelioma ($n=40$)	12/5476 0.2%	78/2187 3.6%	422/10904 3.9%
Total excess	3.7%	15.0%	14.9%

Based mainly on data in A.D. McDonald and J.C. McDonald (1987) Tables 2–3 and 2–4 and in J.C. McDonald and A.D. McDonald (1987) Table 3–3.

More reliable indications of risk are obtained from studies in which attempts have been made to estimate individual exposures in terms of intensity and duration. There are some 11 studies to date in nine population groups which meet this requirement, albeit with exposures based primarily on dust not fibre concentrations and these usually scanty and indifferent in quality. For lung cancer these studies have demonstrated two salient features, evident in Fig. 1.

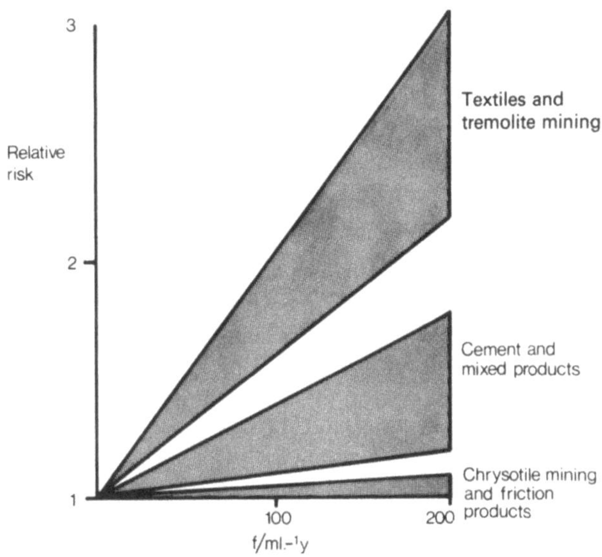

Fig. 1. Relative risk (RR) of lung cancer for different industrial processes and fibre types (see text)

The first is that the exposure-response relationships appear essentially linear and, if expressed as relative risks, pass through the origin. The second is that the gradients vary enormously with both industrial process and fibre type. Thus, the risk of lung cancer from chrysotile exposure is far greater in the manufacture of textiles than of cement or friction products. Similarly, a difference of equal magnitude is exhibited between miners and millers of chrysotile and miners and millers exposed to tremolite. Although the relationships for mesothelioma are less well quantified, higher risks were seen in the same type of industry (e.g. mining, textiles and cement plants) when exposure included amphibole fibres rather than chrysotile alone.

One further epidemiological feature is well established: the risk of lung cancer after asbestos exposure is highly dependent on smoking habit; that of mesothelioma is not. Although, for lung cancer, the interaction appears close to multiplicative (Berry et al. 1985), the number of asbestos workers with lung cancer who have never smoked is small and the histories quite uncertain. On the other hand, if any co-factor is required in mesothelioma it is unlikely to be tobacco (A.D. McDonald and J.C. McDonald 1987).

Linearity – Threshold Issues

The shape of the exposure-response relationship for asbestos-related cancers has considerable academic and scientific importance with great practical and economic implications. When we first reported that there was "a clear direct relationship, which may well be linear, between excess lung cancer mortality and total dust exposure" (Liddell et al. 1977), we had in mind the applications of this finding to the workplace. We gave little thought to the possibility that risk assessments might be attempted by extrapolation to the very much lower airborne fibre concentrations experienced by the general population. Even similar approximations to linearity in further cohort studies did not increase our confidence in the validity of such speculation. We have discussed elsewhere our reasons for questioning this procedure (J.C. McDonald 1985; J.C. McDonald and A.D. McDonald 1987). The main points are as follows:-

1. In all published studies exposure is expressed as the simple product of duration of employment (well documented) and average dust concentration (approximate at best). Bearing in mind the questionable assumption of equivalence between these two components of "cummulative exposure", the remarkable straightness of the lines might be more easily explained by duration of exposure, with little or no contribution from concentration except in quite general terms. The results of an analysis of 58 cases of lung cancer in the Quebec cohort with less than 2 years employment and of 98 referents matched for smoking habit, year of birth, date of employment, gross service and mining area is shown in Table 2 (F.D.K. Liddell and J.C. McDonald, unpublished). Although mean exposure ranged from less than 10

Table 2. Lung cancer in men employed less than 2 years

Concentration (f/ml)	Cases (*n*)	Referents[a] (*n*)	*RR*
< 10	27	44	1
10–29	8	18	0.7
30–99	16	18	1.4
100+	7	18	0.6
	58	98	

[a] Matched for smoking habit, year of birth, date of employment, gross service and mining area.
RR, risk ratio.

to over 100 f/ml no relation to relative risk was seen. Further analyses on these lines are needed to describe the effect on risk of fibre concentration after allowance for duration of exposure.

2. A second general question concerns the comparability of reference populations used in cohort analyses. Figure 2 illustrates the difficulty of detecting whether or not the 11 available fitted lines for exposure response show evidence of a threshold. SMRs at zero exposure range from about 0.5 to over 1.5 and none of the lines pass through the origin. The explanation of this anomaly is presumably that the reference populations are not comparable.
3. A third consideration is the effect of errors and bias both in exposure assessment and in death certification. The first will tend to increase risks at

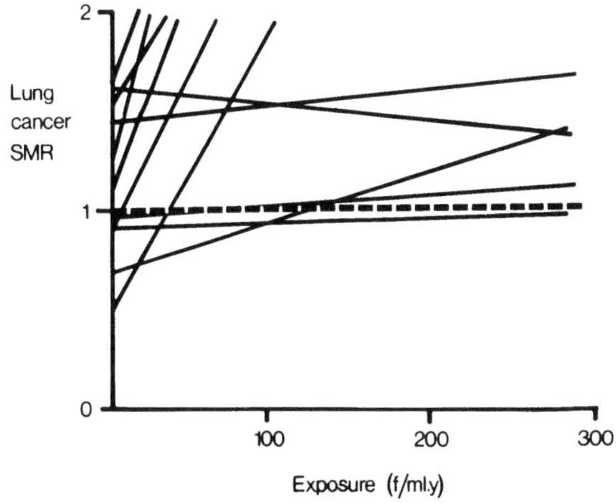

Fig. 2. Standardized mortality ratio (*SMR*) by exposures to asbestos fibres. Exposure-response relationships from 11 studies (see text)

low exposures and decrease them at high exposures (Armstrong, this volume); it will also smooth curves and obscure thresholds. Diagnostic bias in occupational disease can be considerable; in the Quebec study autopsy rates correlated with exposure and may well have influenced the discovery of lung cancers (McDonald et al. 1971). It is also likely that physicians tend to suspect and make appropriate diagnoses in patients known to have had long and heavy dust exposures, and the converse.

4. Finally, it is hard to believe that physiological defence and repair mechanisms are without effect. Such mechanisms must surely prevent or reduce disease at low dust concentrations yielding an effective threshold or at least a sigmoid form of exposure response of the kind familiar to experimental toxicologists.

The same arguments apply to mesothelioma, although here there are no data on the form of relationship to exposure. Nevertheless, these tumours because of their highly specific relationship to asbestos and distinctive clinical and pathological features, provide a valuable measure of environmental impact. During the past 20 or more years the patterns of incidence in Canada, the USA, Britain and Scandinavia have been very similar. Mortality attributed to this disease has increased steeply in men but remained unchanged in women. As there have certainly been some cases in women resulting from occupational or domestic exposure, the absence of any increase over many years in these large industrial populations is remarkable. It implies that cases due to low level exposure unrelated to occupation are too few to be detectable.

The Textiles Anomaly

Although differences in lung cancer risk in the lower two zones of Fig. 1 could conceivably be explained by chance, measurement errors and various local factors, it is most unlikely that those in the upper zone could be. Aside from the cohort of vermiculite miners exposed to fibrous tremolite, where fibre type was a major factor, the remaining four cohorts in the high risk zone were of textile workers. One of these was in England and the other three in the USA. Two of the latter, separately drawn from the same plant in Charleston, South Carolina, were investigated by Dement et al. (1982) and ourselves (McDonald et al. 1983) with closely similar results. At the relevant period, i.e. until the 1950s, chrysotile was the only type of fibre used, mostly obtained from Thetford Mines, Quebec, where the lung cancer risk was very much lower (McDonald et al. 1980). In discussing these findings (McDonald et al. 1983), we stated that "if cocarcinogens can be discounted the cause of this phenomenon must be in the nature of the chrysotile exposure". We had in mind errors in exposure estimation and, in particular, differences in the distribution of very fine long fibres.

We have now completed an investigation of this problem, based on analysis by transmission electron microscopy of nearly 200 lung tissue samples taken at autopsy, half from the Charleston cohort and half from Thetford Mines (Sébastien et al. 1989). Time variables, including duration of employment and interval from last employment to death, were important to this study as was the need to consider chrysotile and tremolite fibres separately. The results showed that neither differences in fibre dimensions nor errors in exposure estimation could explain the anomalous mortality findings. Thus, the question of cocarcinogens cannot be excluded. In particular, the role of mineral oil spray, used widely in American textile plants until the mid 1950s to control dust and facilitate fibre processing, warrants consideration. It will be difficult to investigate this hypothesis epidemiologically, but it might be possible with laboratory animals.

The Tremolite Factor

Tremolite is a mineral silicate which in fibrous and non-fibrous habit is widespread on the earth's surface. It commonly occurs in association with other mineral deposits, some of which are exploited commercially and others not. "Asbestiform" tremolite, as defined by aspect ratio, has occasionally been used for its fibrous qualities and is thus an amphibole asbestos. It is an irregular, but sometimes major, contaminant of many industrial talcs and was suspected many years ago as the factor responsible for lung cancer and mesothelioma in New York State talc miners (Kleinfeld et al. 1967). Trace amounts of tremolite are known to contaminate Quebec chrysotile deposits, especially in the Thetford Mines region. Gibbs (1979) referred to the possibility that talc and associated tremolite might explain the higher frequency of pleural changes, especially calcification, in the chest radiographs of mine workers in Thetford than in Asbestos. The potential importance of fibrous tremolite in the lungs of Quebec chrysotile workers was noted also by Pooley (1976) and Rowlands et al. (1982). Finally, clear evidence of the hazards in terms of exposure response, radiographically and on mortality, was obtained from studies of vermiculite miners and millers in Montana whose only mineral fibre exposure was to contaminating tremolite (McDonald et al. 1986). In 1983 and subsequently, Churg (1987) presented evidence of the predominating presence of tremolite in the lungs of workers and residents of Thetford Mines. He also suggested that tremolite might be important in the genesis of mesothelioma.

Against this background can be considered the findings in our own autopsy survey in chrysotile textile and production workers, mentioned above (Sébastien et al. 1989), and of a recently completed case-referent study of Canadian cases of mesothelioma (McDonald et al. 1989). In the former we observed that although chrysotile comprised about 98.5% of airborne fibres in Thetford Mines and perhaps 99.5% in Charleston, the concentrations of tremolite fibres in lung tissue were higher than of chrysotile in both autopsy series. Table 3 shows that the tremolite/chrysotile ratio increased steadily in both locations with increasing time between end of employment and death. In

Table 3. Tremolite-chrysotile (T/C) ratios in lung at autopsy

Last employment to death (years)	Textile workers ($n=72$)		Miners and millers ($n=89$)	
	mpcf. years	T/C	mpcf. years	T/C
< 1	34	0.5	124	2.7
1–9	53	1.8	579	3.8
10–19	3	2.0	772	5.4
20+	1	n.m.	33	7.8

n.m., not measurable.

our second survey, lung tissue was analysed from 78 cases of mesothelioma in Canada, 1980–1984, and from matched referents. The findings indicated that long amphibole fibres ($\geqq 8\,\mu$m) could explain most of the cases and chrysotile very few. The analysis of short fibres ($\leqq 8\,\mu$m) did not provide additional information. Fibrous tremolite, second only to amosite in apparent importance, appeared responsible for most cases from the Quebec mining region and perhaps one-fifth of those elsewhere. The question which research must now address is the proportion of occupational and non-occupational cases caused by fibrous tremolite and the various possible sources of these fibres. While the latter include chrysotile, vermiculite, talc and several other minerals used in industry, non-industrial sources of air pollution, resulting from wind and water erosion, have also to be considered.

Manmade Mineral Fibres

Early hopes that MMMF – mineral or rock wool and glass fibres or filaments – would eventually replace asbestos for many uses, but without the attendant risks, were shaken in April 1982. In that year, the results of two very large multicentre cohort studies in Europe and the USA, and of a small study in Ontario, were presented at an international symposium in Copenhagen. Quite small increases in standardized mortality ratios (SMRs) for lung cancer were evident 20 or more years after first employment in MMMF production plants and more clearly after 30 years. The similarity of the European and American results was particularly striking (McDonald 1984).

In 1986, an update on all three cohorts was also presented in Copenhagen; the findings now based on larger numbers were again quite similar (see Table 4). In his peer review, Doll (1987) concluded that there was indeed evidence of increased risk of lung cancer, but not of mesothelioma or other disease, greater in the mineral wool than glass wool sector, and mainly in persons employed in the early days of the industry. He noted, however, that several carcinogens could have contributed to the risk and that it was impossible to draw firm quantitative conclusions on dose-response.

Table 4. Lung cancer mortality in American and European cohorts of manmade mineral fiber (MMMF) production workers – summary of findings in 1982 and 1986

	Latency ≧20 years					
	Glass wool/filament			Mineral/rock wool		
	O		E	O		E
To 1982	148		138.7	53		34.5
SMR		1.07			1.54	
1982–86	154		108.8	26		20.7
SMR		1.41			1.26	
To 1986	302		247.5	79		55.2
SMR		1.22			1.43	

Based on McDonald (1984) and Doll (1987).
SMR, standardized mortality ratio; O, observed; E, expected.

The cloud of suspicion that now hangs over the MMMF industry will not be easy to substantiate or dispel. Exposure levels even in the early days of production were probably, by asbestos standards, extremely low and poorly documented. More conclusive evidence might be obtained from workers exposed at much higher levels, for example, men employed on insulation work, were it not that such work has also entailed the probability of high and unmeasured exposure to asbestos, the effects of which cannot be assessed. Electron microscopic studies of lung burden could conceivably provide a way of resolving this problem; however, preliminary results from an ongoing study of lung tissue from former MMMF workers are not promising (P. Sébastien et al., unpublished).

Conclusion

The epidemiological patterns of mesothelioma and lung cancer, as related to mineral fibres, are increasingly distinct. It seems likely that any type of mineral fibre inspired in sufficient quantity over sufficient time may increase the risk of lung cancer in a more or less linear fashion, at least over the middle part of the exposure range. More research is needed to clarify the form of the relationship at very low and very high airborne fibre concentrations. An experimental or sigmoid type of response is biologically plausible and not incompatible with the findings to date, but further statistical analyses are urgently needed to test this hypothesis. Whether mineral fibres are capable of causing lung cancer in the absence of a primary carcinogen such as cigarette smoke remains uncertain; the synergistic action of some co-factor could well explain the high risks experienced by asbestos textile workers.

In contrast to lung cancer, the indications are that the etiology of mesothelioma does not require a co-factor. However, it is clear that mineral fibres differ widely in their capacity to induce this tumour. Man-made fibres have so far not proved able to do so and the same may be true of *pure* chrysotile. On the other hand, there is abundant epidemiological evidence to incriminate the fibrous amphiboles – crocidolite, tremolite and amosite. There are good reasons why these and also erionite fibres (IARC 1987) have this capacity. Fibres in the most carcinogenic size range are not only able, for aerodynamic reasons, to penetrate deeply and reach the pleura but are also extremely resistant to destruction and removal.

These general hypotheses, if correct, have important practical implications. Exposure to any respirable mineral fibres should be kept to a minimum and the use of amphibole and other similar fibres very strictly controlled. The contamination of any mineral used commercially by fibrous tremolite is a potential hazard. Ways need to be found by which otherwise useful products can be monitored and this type of fibre contamination reduced or removed.

References

Berry G, Newhouse ML, Antonis P (1985) Combined effects of asbestos and smoking on mortality from lung cancer and mesothelioma in factory workers. Br J Ind Med 42: 12–18

Churg A (1987) Pathologic reactions to chrysotile and their mineralogic correlates. In: Wagner JC (ed) The biological effects of chrysotile. Lippincott, Philadelphia, pp 54–58

Dement JM, Harris RL, Symons MJ, Shy C (1982) Estimate of dose-response for respiratory cancer among chrysotile asbestos workers. Ann Occup Hyg 26: 869–887

Doll R (1987) Symposium on MMMF, Copenhagen, October 1986: Overview and conclusions. Ann Occp Hyg 31: 805–819

Doll R, Peto J (1987) Other asbestos-related neoplasms. In: Antman K, Aisner J (eds) Asbestos-related malignancy. Grune and Stratton, London, pp 81–96

Gibbs GW (1979) Etiology of pleural calcification: a study of Quebec chrysotile asbestos miners and millers. Arch Environ Health 34: 76–83

IARC: International Agency for Research on Cancer (1987) Silica and some Silicates. IARC, Lyon, pp 225–239

IARC monographs on the evaluation of the carcinogenic risk of chemicals to humans, vol 42.

Kleinfeld M, Messite J, Kooyman O, Zaki MH (1967) Mortality among talc miners and millers in New York State. Arch Environ Health 14: 663–667

Liddell FDK (1988) The possible link between exposure to asbestos and laryngeal cancer. Report to Industrial Injuries Advisory Council (UK), 29 Feb 1988

Liddell FDK, McDonald JC, Thomas DC (1977) Methods of cohort analysis: appraisal by application to asbestos mining. J R Stat Soc A 140: 469–491

McDonald AD, McDonald JC (1987) Epidemiology of malignant mesothelioma. In: Antman K, Aisner J (eds) Asbestos-related malignancy. Grune and Stratton, London, pp 31–55

McDonald AD, Fry JS, Woolley AD, McDonald JC (1983) Dust exposure and mortality in an American chrysotile textile plant. Br J Ind Med 40: 361–367

McDonald JC (1984) Peer review: mortality of workers exposed to MMMF – current evidence and future research. In: Guthe T (ed) Biological effects of man-made mineral fibres, vol 1. WHO Europe, Copenhagen, pp 369–380
McDonald JC (1985) Health implications of environmental exposure to asbestos. Environ Health Perspect 62: 319–328
McDonald JC, McDonald AD (1987) Epidemiology of asbestos-related lung cancer. In: Antman K, Aisner J (eds) Asbestos-related malignancy. Grune and Stratton, London, pp 57–79
McDonald JC, McDonald AD, Gibbs GW, Siemiatycki J, Rossiter CE (1971) Mortality in the chrysotile asbestos mines and mills of Quebec. Arch Environ Health 22: 677–686
McDonald JC, Liddell FDK, Gibbs GW, Eyssen GE, McDonald AD (1980) Dust exposure and mortality in chrysotile mining, 1910–75. Br J Ind Med 37: 11–24
McDonald JC, McDonald AD, Armstrong B, Sébastien P (1986) Cohort study of mortality in vermiculite miners exposed to tremolite. Br J Ind Med 43: 436–444
McDonald JC, Armstrong B, Case B, Doell D, McCaughey WTE, McDonald AD, Sébastien P (1989) Mesothelioma and asbestos fibre type: evidence from lung tissue analyses. Cancer 63: 1544–1547
Pooley FD (1976) An examination of the fibrous mineral content of lung tissue from the Canadian chrysotile mining industry. Environ Res 12: 281–298
Rowlands N, Gibbs GW, McDonald AD (1982) Asbestos fibres in the lungs of chrysotile miners and millers – a preliminary report 26: 411–415
Sébastien P, McDonald JC, McDonald AD, Case B, Harley R (1989) Respiratory cancer in chrysotile textile and mining industries: exposure inferences from lung analysis. Br J Ind Med 46: 180–187

Herbicides and Cancer: A Review and Discussion of Methodologic Issues

A. Blair and S. Hoar Zahm

Occupational Studies Section, National Cancer Institute, Bethesda, MD 208 92, USA

In the late 1970s and early 1980s, investigators in Sweden reported over fivefold risks for soft-tissue sarcoma and lymphoma among persons exposed to phenoxyacetic acid herbicides and chlorophenols (Eriksson et al. 1981; Hardell and Sandstrom 1979; Hardell et al. 1981). The possibility that these widely used and important commercial chemicals might be human carcinogens prompted a number of epidemiologic investigations. Reports from over 20 additional studies are now available. Results from these investigations, which employed cohort and case-control designs, have not been consistent, but as of yet the discrepancies cannot be explained. The purpose of this paper is to provide a brief overview of available findings, to note consistencies and inconsistencies, to consider methodologic issues, particularly for case-control studies that might account for these inconsistencies, and to identify areas of research needing development.

Completed Studies

Descriptions of studies designed to evaluate cancer risks from occupational exposure to herbicides are included in Table 1. We have chosen not to include evaluations of Vietnam veterans because for most their manner of exposure differs from farmers and industrial workers. Cohort studies, which have included both manufacturers and applicators, have usually evaluated all causes of death. Most, however, have lacked sufficient power to adequately evaluate small to moderate risks for rare tumors. Case-control studies have focused primarily on soft-tissue sarcomas (STS), Hodgkin's disease (HD), and non-Hodgkin's lymphoma (NHL), but single studies have been completed on multiple myeloma (MM), ovarian mesothelioma, sinonasal cancer (SNC), and nasopharyngeal cancer (NPC). Exposed subjects in the case-control studies have been predominantly farmers and foresters.

Results for selected cancers from the completed studies are summarized in Table 2. A striking feature is the considerable variation in the estimates of relative risks. For STS, estimates range from over fivefold to slight deficits,

Recent Results in Cancer Research, Vol. 120

although 8 of the 13 studies have relative risks greater than 1.0. The largest relative risks for STS occurred in the initial studies from Sweden (Eriksson et al. 1981; Hardell and Sandstrom 1979), but at least twofold excesses also occurred in recent case-control studies of women in Italy (Vineis et al. 1987) and men in Sweden (Hardell and Eriksson 1988). Over twofold excesses have been reported in two cohort studies (Kauppinen et al. 1986; Lynge 1985). However, only one death occurred from STS in a U.S. cohort of manufacturers (Ott et al. 1987) and only one of five cases worked in the phenoxyacetic acid manufacturing department in the Danish cohort (Lynge 1985). The authors of the Danish study, however, suspect others may have had some exposure to herbicides, particularly the three cases who worked in the shipping department (Lynge 1985).

Lymphatic and hematopoietic cancers have been evaluated frequently with NHL and HD receiving particular attention. Except for the Swedish findings (Hardell et al. 1981), where a fivefold risk occurred, the pattern for HD is unimpressive. Excesses of NHL among groups exposed to phenoxyacetic acid herbicides have been reported in cohort and case-control studies. As with STS, the range in relative risks for NHL is considerable (from 3.9 to a deficit of 0.4). In studies from Sweden (Hardell et al. 1981) and Kansas (Hoar et al. 1986), the risk of NHL rose considerably with the number of days herbicides were used. In a cohort study of manufacturers in the U.S. (Bond et al. 1988), the two deaths from NHL occurred among men who were employed in the 2,4-D plant, while none were associated with other production processes. These two workers had also been employed in other departments.

Risks for multiple myeloma (MM) and leukemia show consistent elevations, but the numbers are small. A threefold excess of multiple myeloma and lymphatic cancers other than lymphosarcoma and HD among manufacturers (Bond et al. 1988), however, indicates that these cancers deserve further evaluation.

Excesses of lung, stomach, and prostate cancer have occurred in several cohort studies of manufacturers and applicators. Case-control studies of these tumors have not been conducted where the objective was to evaluate risks from herbicides. Stomach and prostate cancer are of particular interest given these cancers are often elevated among farmers (Blair et al. 1985). Many farmers also come into contact with herbicides, although dietary factors and other lifestyle factors could also be involved. Farmers, for example, smoke less than many other occupational groups, which probably accounts for their generally low rates for lung cancer (Blair et al. 1985). The 17-fold excess of lung cancer among Finnish woodworkers (Kauppinen et al. 1986) may be due to exposure to such items as wood dust, arsenic, or chromates, although they also had exposure to pesticides. The excesses for ovarian mesothelioma (Donna et al. 1984), nasopharyngeal and sinonasal cancer (Hardell et al. 1982), and testicular cancer (Bond et al. 1988; Coggon et al. 1986) were in only one or two studies and need further evaluation. These cancers have not received as much attention as STS, HDL, and HD, particularly in case-control studies, but the excesses noted indicate that additional evaluation is needed.

Table 1. Description of completed studies on cancer and herbicides

Reference	Study design	Population/ location	Years covered	Number of subjects[a]	Cancers	Exposure based on	Herbicides mentioned
Hardell and Sandstrom (1979)	Ca-co	N. Sweden	1970–1979	52/206	STS	Interviews	Phenoxys; chlorophenols
Eriksson et al. (1981)	Ca-co	S. Sweden	1974–1978	110/220	STS	Interviews	Phenoxys; chlorophenols
Smith et al. (1984)	Ca-co	New Zealand	1976–1980	82/92	STS	Interviews	Primarily 2,4,5-T
Smith and Pearce (1986)	Ca-co	New Zealand	1976–1980	51/315	STS	Interviews	Primarily 2,4,5-T
Vineis et al. (1987)	Ca-co	Italy	1981–1983	68/158	STS	Interviews	2,4,5-T; 2,4,-D; MCPA
Hardell and Eriksson (1988)	Ca-co	Sweden	1978–1983	54/321	STS	Interviews	Phenoxys; chlorophenols
Hardell et al. (1981)	Ca-co	Sweden	1974–1978	169/338	NHL, HD	Interviews	2,4,5-T; 2,4-D; MCPA
Hoar et al. (1986)	Ca-co	Kansas	1976–1982	424/948	NHL, HD, STS	Interviews	Primarily 2,4-D
Pearce et al. (1986a)	Ca-co	New Zealand	1977–1981	83/228	NHL	Interviews	Primarily 2,4,5-T
Pearce et al. (1987)	Ca-co	New Zealand	1977–1981	183/396	NHL	Interviews	Primarily 2,4,5-T
Woods et al. (1987)	Ca-co	Washington	1981–1984	499/694	STS, NHL	Interviews	Phenoxys; chlorophenols
Pearce et al. (1986b)	Ca-co	New Zealand	1977–1981	76/315	MM	Interviews	Primarily 2,4,5-T
Hardell et al. (1982)	Ca-co	Sweden	1970–1979	71/541	SNC, NPC	Interviews	Phenoxys; amitrol
Donna et al. (1984)	Ca-co	Italy	1974–1980	60/127	Ovarian mesothelioma	Interviews	Unspecified
Axelson et al. (1980)	Cohort	Railroad workers	1957–1978	348	All causes	Job titles	Phenoxys; amitrol; diuron
Zack and Suskind (1980)	Cohort	Manufacturers	1949–1978	121	All causes	Chloracne	2,4,5-T
Theiss et al. (1982)	Cohort	Manufacturers	1953–1979	70	All causes	Accident	2,4,5-T
Riihimaki et al. (1982)	Cohort	Applicators	1955–1980	1971	All causes	Job title	2,4,5-T; 2,4-D
Lynge (1985)	Cohort	Manufacturers	1947–1982	4459	All cancers	Job title	2,4,5-T; 2,4-D; MCPA
Coggon et al. (1986)	Cohort	Manufacturers	1947–1983	5784	All causes	Job title	Mostly MCPA
Kauppinen et al. (1986)	Cohort	Woodworkers	1957–1980	3805	Respiratory cancers	Job title	Chlorophenols, arsenic

Ott et al. (1987)	Cohort	Manufacturers	1940–1982	2187	All causes	Job title and monitoring data	Primarily 2,4,5-T; mostly phenoxys
Wiklund et al. (1987)	Cohort	Applicators	1965–1982	20245	NHL, HD		
Bond et al. (1988)	Cohort	Manufacturers	1945–1982	878	All causes	Job title	Mostly 2,4-D

[a] Number of cases and controls for case-control studies, or number of subjects in cohort studies.
Ca-co, case-control.

Table 2. Risks for selected cancers from phenoxyacid herbicide exposure

Reference	Study	Cancer (relative risks (no. of exposed cases))									
	Design	STS	NHL	HD	MM	Leukemia	Lung	Stomach	Esophagus	Prostate	Ovary or testis
Hardell and Sandstrom (1979)	Ca-co	5.3*(13)									
Eriksson et al. (1981)	Ca-co	6.8*(14)									
Smith et al. (1984)	Ca-co	1.3(21)									
Smith and Pearce (1986)	Ca-co	0.7(6)									
Hoar et al. (1986)	Ca-co	1.4(15)[f]	2.2*(24)[f]	1.0(13)[f]							
Woods et al. (1987)	Ca-co	0.8[j]	1.1[j]								
Vineis et al. (1987)	Ca-co	2.4(4)[k]									
Hardell and Eriksson (1988)	Ca-co	3.3*(9)									
Hardell et al. (1981)	Ca-co		4.8*(41)[a]								
Pearce et al. (1986a)	Ca-co		1.6(51)[p]								
Pearce et al. (1987)	Ca-co		1.0(72)								
Pearce et al. (1986b)	Ca-co				1.3(43)						

Table 2 (*continued*)

Reference	Study	Cancer (relative risks (no. of exposed cases))									
	Design	STS	NHL	HD	MM	Leukemia	Lung	Stomach	Esophagus	Prostate	Ovary or testis
Donna et al. (1984)	Ca-co										4.4(18)[o]
Axelson et al. (1980)	Cohort						–(0)	3.1(2)			
Zack and Suskind (1980)	Cohort		3.4(3)[b]				2.8(5)	–(0)			
Theiss et al. (1982)	Cohort	–(0)	–(0)[b]				2.4(3)	4.3(3)			
Riihimaki et al. (1982)	Cohort				5.0(1)[e]		1.1(12)[e]	1.1[c]		1.8(2)[e]	
Lynge (1985)	Cohort	2.7(5)[l]	1.3(7)[a]			1.1(5)[l]	1.2(38)[l]	1.3(12)[l]	1.7(3)[l]	0.8(9)[l]	
Coggon et al. (1986)	Cohort	1.0(1)	0.4(2)	0.3(1)[l]	1.6(5)	1.8(14)	1.2(117)	0.9(26)	0.9(8)	1.3(18)	2.2(4)[n]
Kauppinen et al. (1986)	Cohort						17.4*(4)[d]			1.9(8)[d]	
Ott et al. (1987)	Cohort	2.5(1)	1.9(5)	0.9(1)	2.0(2)	1.2(4)	0.8(23)	1.6(6)[d]		1.9(8)	
Wiklund et al. (1987)	Cohort		1.0(21)	1.2(11)							
Bond et al. (1988)	Cohort	–(0)	3.9(2)[m]	2.6(1)	3.1(5)[i]	2.2(2)	1.0(8)	–(0)	–(0)	1.0(1)	4.6(1)[n]

* $P < =0.05$
[a] NHL and HD.
[b] Lymphatic and hematopoietic cancer.
[c] Stomach and esophagus cancer with 10-year latency.
[d] Respiratory cancer with 5 years of exposure.
[e] > 9-year latency.
[f] Used 2,4-D.
[g] Chronic lymphatic and acute myeloid leukemia exposed to 2,4-D.
[i] Other lymphatic and hematopoietic cancer.
[j] Number exposed not provided.
[k] Women only.
[l] Men only.
[m] Lymphosarcoma and reticulosarcoma.
[n] Testis.
[o] Ovarian cancer
[p] Using general population controls.

The most striking feature of the results from these reports is the inconsistency. Inconsistency is not an uncommon feature of epidemiologic studies, but it typically occurs when some studies show a small risk and others show none at all. It is unusual, however, for situations to occur where the estimates vary as widely as they do for some cancers (i.e., from none to over fivefold) among persons exposed to herbicides. Various explanations might account for these discrepancies, including study design, type of exposure (2,4,5-T, MCPA, or 2,4-D), level of exposure (the shorter spray season in Sweden may result in a more intense exposure than in other areas; Woods et al. 1987), level and type of contaminants such as dioxins and dibenzofurans which may differ by chemical and/or by country, effect modification by occupational or other exposures, susceptibility of the populations studied, exposure and/or disease misclassification, small numbers, and random error. To date, however, no explanation appears fully satisfactory.

Methodologic Issues

Space does not permit a detailed evaluation of the strengths and weaknesses of each of the completed studies. Many, however, are high quality investigations with sufficient power to detect moderate risks for some cancers. Several case-control studies were population-based and incorporated important methodologic strengths such as pathologic review of diagnoses, inclusion of cancers supposedly unrelated to herbicide exposure as a special set of controls, and attempts to corroborate subject's reports of herbicide use. For example, the case-control studies showing striking positive associations between NHL and herbicides from Sweden (Hardell et al. 1981) and Kansas (Hoar et al. 1986) and those showing little association from New Zealand (Pearce et al. 1986a) and Washington (Woods et al. 1987) are all of a population-based, interview design. Although some of the cohort studies were too small to evaluate risks for rare cancers, most have excellent documentation of exposure (either from plant job history records or the development of chloracne). In short, there appear to be no obvious methodologic differences that distinguish the highly positive studies from the others.

Exposure evaluation is always a major concern in epidemiologic studies and exposure misclassification has been raised as a possible explanation for the discrepancies noted in Table 2. Historical assessment of occupational exposures from interviews is difficult, but evaluation of exposure to herbicides may be particularly problematic because of their relatively infrequent use by most subjects.

Exposure evaluation in case-control studies based on interviews is more suspect than from cohort studies where records are available. Case-control studies have played a prominent role in the issue of herbicides and cancer, therefore, problems associated with assessment of herbicide in case-control studies deserve special attention. Since several case-control investigations have employed methods similar to those used in Kansas (Hoar et al. 1986), we will use results from this case-control study of STS, NHL, and HD to evaluate general limitations of exposure evaluation associated with this study design and to assess their potential influence on risk estimates.

The essential findings of the Kansas study are shown in Table 3. Briefly, NHL was associated with reported use of herbicides by farmers, but STS and HD were not. For NHL, the risk rose with number of days per year of herbicide use, was greater among those who mixed or applied herbicides themselves, among those who used backpack sprayers, or among those who did not use protective equipment, and was most strongly associated with those who reported they used 2,4-D. Risks were similar when use was based on information from interviews of subjects or next-of-kin and the association could not be accounted for by other factors such as insecticide use, other occupational exposures, family history of cancer, medical conditions, or medical treatments. NHL was associated with the number of years of herbicide use, but the association disappeared

Table 3. Odds ratios (ORs) from herbicide exposure in the Kansas study. (Hoar et al 1986)

Factor	Relative risks						
Herbicide	ORs for NHL, HD, and STS were 0.9, 0.9, and 1.6, respectively						
Frequency (days per year)		0 Days	1–5 Days	6–10 Days	11–20 Days	< 20 Days	*P* for trend
of herbicide exposure	NHL	1.0	1.4	1.6	2.6	6.0*	0.0004
	HD	1.0	1.0	0.4	1.3	1.0	0.29
	STS	1.0	0.6	0.5	2.9	0.8	0.50
For NHL only							
Days of herbicide use among those reporting 2,4-D exposure		1.0	1.6	1.9	3.0	7.6*	0.0001
Mixers/applicators	Yes, OR = 1.9; No, OR = 1.1						
Mixer/applicator by days of exposure per year		1.0	1.4	1.5	1.8	8.0*	
Protective equipment	Yes, OR = 1.5, No, OR = 2.1						
Backpack or hand sprayers	OR = 2.3						
Type of phenoxyacid	2,4-D only: OR = 2.6; 2,4,5-T (most had 2,4-D use): OR = 1.2						
Herbicide exposure by vital status	Deceased, OR = 1.5; Living, OR = 1.7						
	Deceased with long-term use, OR = 5.5; living with long-term use, OR = 5.6						
Supplier's corroboration	Use verified, OR = 1.8; interview data only, OR = 1.6						

* $P < = 0.05$.

when adjusted for number of days of use. These data will be used to illustrate general methodologic issues surrounding case-control studies of cancer and herbicides such as power, diagnosis of cancers of primary interest (lymphatic and hematopoietic cancer and soft-tissue sarcomas), and exposure evaluation and likely affect on risk estimates.

Power

The first epidemiologic study noting an association between cancer and herbicides was from a small case-control study of STS (52 cases) (Hardell and Sandstrom 1979). Subsequent case-control studies of this and other cancers, however, have been larger, ranging from 80 to over 200 cases, depending upon the tumor of interest. These studies typically were large enough to detect excess risks from two- to three-fold, depending upon the definition of exposure. The Kansas study (Hoar et al. 1986), with 130 to 170 cases (depending upon the cancer) and over 900 controls, is one of the larger investigations.

Some reviewers of these studies have pointed out that the odds ratios (ORs) for most exposure subcategories (such as days per year of use), are based on small numbers and they are generally not statistically significant. Numbers of subjects in the subcategories are small compared with the entire data set. For example, in the Kansas study there were seven cases of NHL and 12 controls reporting use of herbicides 20 or more days per year. In exposure-response analyses, however, the test for trend is the critical test for an exposure-response gradient because it uses all subjects and weights the test for significance by the number of subjects in each category. This test is much more powerful than any single category comparison. Confidence intervals also provide guidance in evaluating risks based on small numbers. Finally, small numbers in exposure-response categories would introduce variability in risk estimates and such variability would be as likely to destroy exposure-response gradients as to create them. In studies where exposure-response trends occur, it seems unlikely that such patterns would be caused by the reduction in numbers in the strata. In the Kansas study, the trend by days per year of use was highly significant and the 95% confidence interval for the NHL risk ratio associated with $\geq$ 20 days per year of herbicide use, although broad (from 1.9 to 19.5), has a lower bound that is clearly above 1.0.

Case Definition and Diagnosis

Diagnosis of STS and NHL is difficult. STS includes a heterogeneous group of cancers and the definition of STS varied by study. The studies in Sweden (Eriksson et al. 1981; Hardell and Sandstrom 1979) and Kansas (Hoar et al. 1986) included soft-tissue tumors at all sites while some other studies included only those designated by the ICDA code 171. The studies in Sweden and

Table 4. Exposure issues in case-control studies of cancer and herbicides

Issue	Probable effect on OR	Comment
Nonrandom response bias		
Better recall by cases	Overestimate	If operating, this recall bias must have been restricted to NHL cases, since ORs for HD and STS were not elevated in the Kansas study (Hoar et al. 1986). Similarity, no significant excess of colon cancer was found in Sweden (Hardell 1981). The survey of suppliers found no differences in corroboration between cases and controls suggesting case response bias did not occur (Hoar et al. 1986)
Random misclassification		
Inaccurate recall of herbicide by all subjects	Underestimate	Recall problems clearly occurred since agreement between subjects and suppliers was about 50%. It is not obvious, however, which report was more accurate. In any case, such misclassification would diminish exposure-response associations
Inaccurate recall of specific herbicides used	Underestimate	NHL ORs for the >20 days of use category increase as specificity of exposure increases (OR for herbicides in general=6.0, but for those using 2,4-D=8.6)
Interviews of next-of-kin who may not know the subject's history of herbicide use well	Underestimate	NHL ORs for the 20 or more days per year category were similar whether based on interviews of subjects themselves (OR=5.6) or next-of-kin (OR=5.5)
Small percentage of subjects exposed to herbicides	Underestimate	The percentage may be too low, however, study subjects are elderly and many may have farmed before herbicides were widely used. Our definition for farmers also included subjects who may have only lived on farms during childhood and may never have actually engaged in farm activities
Risk not related to acres treated	Underestimate	Acres treated may be a poorer measure of exposure than days per year of use and this would account for the lack of association with this measure. Larger operations may use more efficient equipment and, thus, acres treated may not reflect days of use. The EPA has found that the number of acres treated is not positively associated with level of 2,4-D in the urine (EPA 1985). In any case, even if acres treated was a more accurate measure of exposure, this would not cause a positive exposure-response gradient for days per year. If days per year

		was a poorer measure of exposure than acres treated, then random misclassification should occur which would lower risk estimates associated with this measure
Farmers do not use herbicides 20 or more days per year	Underestimate	NHL exposure-response gradient by days per year would be even steeper than noted, resulting in higher risks at lower exposure levels than reported
Other issues		
Could not link risk to days per year for 2,4-D specifically	Underestimate	Correct. This, however, implies misclassification of days per year of use for 2,4-D with some other herbicide which would depress risk estimates for 2,4-D
Little association with duration of use	— — —	In this study, duration meant years of use on the farm, and years of herbicide use would not be as relevant as years of personal use. Duration is probably not as accurate a measure of exposure to herbicides as days per year because these chemicals are used only a few days per year by most farmers
Risks not specific to histology subtypes or grade	Under- or overestimate	Difficulties in classification of subtypes of NHL would tend to minimize subgroup difference (Dick et al. 1987) by depressing estimates of risks for subtypes strongly associated with herbicides and increasing risks for other subtypes
Only OR in the > 20 days per year category was significant	— — —	A trend test is the more powerful, and the more appropriate, measure of effect
Association due to confounding from other factors	Under- or overestimate risks	The study results were directly adjusted for other pesticide use, radiation, medical conditions and treatment, and other occupational factors. Few strong risk factors for NHL are known and they would have to be similar in magnitude and parallel herbicide exposure to effect the exposure-response relationship

OR, odds ratio.

Kansas, therefore, may include a more heterogeneous group of cancers than other studies which would tend to mute estimates of relative risks. Inclusion of cancers which may have different etiologies might, therefore, be a partial explanation for the lack of an association between STS and herbicides in Kansas. It would not, however, explain the positive association with NHL in Kansas, nor with NHL and STS in Sweden.

Classification of histologic subtypes of NHL is also difficult, particularly when based on morphologic aspects discernable using the light microscope (Dick et al. 1987). In studies in Sweden (Eriksson et al. 1981; Hardell and Sandstrom 1979; Hardell et al. 1981), Kansas (Hoar et al. 1986), Italy (Vineis et al. 1987), and Washington (Woods et al. 1987), pathologic tissues received special review by panels of pathologists. In the Kansas study (Hoar et al. 1986), about 20% of the original STS cases were excluded following the review. These special reviews would minimize, but not eliminate, diagnostic misclassification. They would, however, result in a more consistent definition of disease within a study and would reduce variations in diagnoses by calendar time or geography which might also be associated with exposure. Any remaining misdiagnosis of cases is likely to be random which would depress risk estimates.

More sophisticated classifications of NHL and STS which can minimize heterogeneous groupings are needed in future studies. In particular, some have suggested that immunologic markers should be included (Dick et al. 1987).

Exposure Evaluation

A major limitation in case-control studies is the accuracy and reliability of exposure assessment (Blair et al. 1989). The problem is particularly severe in studies of chronic diseases such as cancer where the important exposures may have occurred several years or several decades before diagnosis of the disease. The Kansas study (Hoar et al. 1986) can be used to demonstrate and evaluate the impact various problems associated with assessment of past exposure to herbicides may have had on risk estimates. Several issues relating to the assessment of herbicide exposure in this study are listed in Table 4, along with their probable effect on risk estimates. Many of these issues are also applicable to other case-control studies listed in Tables 1 and 2.

The items and issues noted in Table 4 underscore the difficulty in assessing pesticide exposure in case-control studies by interview. These issues and criticisms are well founded and do affect estimates of risk. Few, however, would provide explanations for a positive association (case recall bias is an exception). To the contrary, these problems are likely to underestimate the risks, and, thus, to explain the lack of an association between STS and HD and herbicides in the Kansas study, NHL in Washington, or STS and NHL in New Zealand. Case response bias could, of course, create spurious associations, but it did not appear to be operative in our data for two reasons. First, it would have had to be restricted to NHL cases since there was no association with STS and HD, and second, information from the corroborative survey with pesticide suppliers indicated that the level of agreement between subjects and suppliers did not differ between cases and controls. Other studies have also used these techniques to evaluate the potential for case-response bias.

Most of the potential problems in exposure assessment in the Kansas and other studies would, therefore, tend to reduce estimates of relative risk and to mute exposure-response relations. Misclassifications of exposure might be a reasonable explanation for the lack of an association between herbicides and STS and HD in Kansas, but, it cannot explain the strong association with NHL. Likewise, misclassification might be a plausible explanation for the lack of an association between herbicides and cancer in some of the other studies, but it is an unlikely explanation for the positive associations.

Research Needs

The major limitation in conducting case-control, and probably cohort, studies of herbicides and cancer is the difficulty in accurately estimating relevant historical exposures. Persons exposed to pesticides are seldom exposed to single agents and the chemicals of choice for specific pests have changed over the years. These factors create uncertainties, particularly in studies where exposure is based on subject recall. In general, problems in exposure evaluation would bias risk estimates toward the null, however, the problem of concomitant exposures could also result in an excess risk being inappropriate affiliated with a specific pesticide. Although these problems are similar to those experienced by occupational studies in general and by other areas of epidemiologic research, such as diet, relatively little methodologic research has been conducted with respect to pesticides.

With the general lack of historical monitoring data on pesticide exposures, epidemiologists will most likely be forced to continue to rely, to some extent, upon self-reports to assess exposures. Thus, methodologic studies are needed to evaluate a variety of issues, including comparability of interview information on pesticide use obtained (a) from subjects versus next-of-kin, (b) from interviews versus reinterviews, (c) from records versus interviews, (d) from pesticide suppliers versus subjects, and (e) from estimates of level of exposure based on interviews versus those based on monitoring. Additional work is also needed to determine how much information regarding exposure to pesticides may be obtained by interview. To date, interviews have typically obtained the name of the pesticides used, the years of use, some indication of the frequency of use, and whether or not protective equipment was used. There are several reasons why more detailed questions on pesticide use have not been asked, but a major factor has been the belief that respondents would be unable to provide accurate responses. This assumption may be correct for some occupations, but not others. Farmers, for example, may represent a group who may be able to provide detailed information since most are independent businessmen and they must personally decide what pesticide is needed and make the purchase, mix, and apply, or arrange for application. These responsibilities increase the likelihood that they may be able to recall more details on pesticide use than casual pesticide users. Factors that appear to affect level of exposure include the size of containers of concentrated pesticide, the time spent mixing pesticides and repairing equipment, the degree of skin contact, the frequency of washing to remove pesticide from the skin, the frequency of clothing changes, the time delay before entering sprayed fields, and the type of protective equipment used. Methodologic investigations are needed to assess the opportunity of obtaining such information by interview. Methodologic efforts are also needed to evaluate opportunities to supplement information obtained directly from study subjects with data from colleagues and pesticide suppliers, from monitoring of current exposures, from county extension agents, and other sources. Only by collecting information from a variety of sources and evaluating its comparability are we likely to make significant strides in improving exposure evaluation in studies of pesticides.

References

Axelson O, Sundell L, Andersson K, Edling C, Hogstedt C, Kling H (1980) Herbicide exposure and tumor mortality: an updated epidemiologic investigation on Swedish railroad workers. Scand J Work Environ Health 6: 73–79

Blair A, Malker H, Cantor KP, Burmeister L, Wiklund K (1985) Cancer among farmers: a review. Scand J Work Environ Health 11: 397–407

Blair A, Zahm SH, Cantor KP, Stewart PA (1989) Estimating exposure to pesticides in epidemiologic studies of cancer. Am Chem Soc Symp Ser. 382. American Chemical Society, Washington, DC, pp 38–46

Bond GG, Wetterstroem NH, Roush GJ, McLaren EA, Lipps TE, Cook RR (1988) Cause-specific mortality among employees engaged in the manufacture, formulation, or packaging of 2,4-dichlorophenoxyacetic acid and related salts. Br J Ind Med 45: 98–105

Coggon D, Pannett B, Winter PD, Acheson ED, Bonsall J (1986) Mortality of workers exposed to 2 methyl-4 chlorophenoxyacetic acid. Scand J Work Environ Health 12: 448–454

Dick F, Van Lier S, Banks P, Frizzera G, Witrak G, Gibson R, Schuman L, Isacson P, O'Conor G, Cantor K, Blattner W, Blair A (1987) Use of the working formulation for non-Hodgkin's lymphoma in epidemiologic studies: agreement between reported diagnoses and a panel of experimental pathologists. JNCI 78: 1137–1144

Donna A, Betta F, Robutti F, Crosignani P, Berrino F, Bellingeri D (1984) Ovarian mesothelial tumors and herbicides: a case-control study. Carcinogenesis 5: 941–942

EPA: U.S. Environmental Protection Agency (1985) Final report: applicator and mixer/loader exposure to pesticides during ground boom spraying operations. Versar, Springfield Va (EPA contract no 68–01–6271; task no 48)

Eriksson M, Hardell L, Berg NO, Moller T, Axelson O (1981) Soft-tissue sarcoma and exposure to chemical substances: a case-referent study. Br J Ind Med 38: 27–33

Hardell L (1981) Relation of soft-tissue sarcoma, malignant lymphoma, and colon cancer to phenoxyacids, chlorophenols, and other agents. Scand J Work Environ Health 7: 119–130

Hardell L, Sandstrom A (1979) Case-control study: soft-tissue sarcomas and exposure to phenoxyacetic acids or chlorophenols. Br J Cancer 39: 711–717

Hardell L, Eriksson M (1988) The association between soft-tissue sarcomas and exposure to phenoxyacetic acids: a new case-referent study. Cancer 62: 652–656

Hardell L, Eriksson M, Lenner P, Lungren E (1981) Malignant lymphoma and exposure to chemicals especially organic solvents, chlorophenols and phenoxy acids: a case-control study. Br J Cancer 43: 169–176

Hardell L, Johansson B, Axelson O (1982) Epidemiological study of nasal and nasopharyngeal cancer and their relation to phenoxy acid or chlorophenol exposure. Am J Ind Med 3: 247–257

Hoar SK, Blair A, Holmes FF, Boysen CD, Robel RJ, Hoover R, Fraumeni JR Jr (1986) Agricultural herbicide use and risk of lymphoma and soft-tissue sarcoma. JAMA 256: 1141–1147

Kauppinen TP, Partanen TJ, Nurminen MM, Nickels JI, Hernberg SG, Hakulinen TR, Pukkala EI, Savonen ET (1986) Respiratory cancers and chemical exposures in the wood industry: a nested case-control study. Br J Ind Med 43: 84–90

Lynge E (1985) A follow-up study of cancer incidence among workers in manufacture of phenoxy herbicides in Denmark. Br J Cancer 52: 259–270

Ott MG, Olson RA, Cook RR, Bond GG (1987) Cohort mortality study of chemical workers with potential exposure to the higher chlorinated dioxins. J Occup Med 29: 422–429

Pearce NE, Smith AH, Howard JK, Sheppard RA, Giles HJ, Teague CA (1986a) Non-Hodgkin's lymphoma and exposure to phenoxyherbicides, chlorophenols, fencing work, and meat works employment: a case-control study. Br J Ind Med 43: 75–83

Pearce NE, Smith AH, Howard JK, Sheppard RA, Giles HJ, Teague CA (1986b) Case-control study of multiple myeloma and farming. Br J Cancer 54: 493–500

Pearce NE, Sheppard RA, Smith AH, Teague CA (1987) Non-Hodgkin's lymphoma and farming: an expanded case-control study. Int J Cancer 39: 155–161

Riihimaki V, Asp S, Hernberg S (1982) Mortality of 2,4-dichlorophenoxyacetic acid and 2,4,5-trichlorophenoxyacetic acid herbicide applicators in Finland. Scand J Work Environ Health 8: 37–42

Smith AH, Pearce NE (1986) Update on soft tissue sarcoma and phenoxyherbicides in New Zealand. Chemosphere 15: 1795–1798

Smith AH, Pearce NE, Fisher DO, Giles HJ, Teague CA, Howard JK (1984) Soft tissue sarcoma and exposure to phenoxyherbicides and chlorophenols in New Zealand. JNCI 73: 1111–1117

Theiss AM, Frentzel-Beyme R, Link R (1982) Mortality study of persons exposed to dioxin in a trichlorophenol-process accident that occurred in the BASF AG on November 17, 1953. Am J Ind Med 3: 179–189

Vineis P, Terracini B, Ciccone G, Cignetti A, Colombo E, Donna A, Maffi L, Pisa R, Ricci P, Zanini E, Comba P (1987) Phenoxy herbicides and soft-tissue sarcomas in female rice weeders. Scand J Work Environ Health 13: 9–17

Wiklund K, Dich J, Holm LE (1987) Risk of malignant lymphoma in Swedish pesticide appliers. Br J Cancer 56: 505–508

Woods JS, Polissar L, Seveson RK, Heuser LS, Kulander BG (1987) Soft tissue sarcoma and non-Hodgkin's lymphoma in relation to phenoxyherbicide and chlorinated phenol exposure in Western Washington. JNCI 78: 899–910

Zack JA, Suskind RR (1980) The mortality experience of workers exposed to tetrachlorodibenzodioxin in a trichlorophenol process accident. J Occup Med 22: 11–14

Cancer Risks from Exposure to Radon Progeny in Mines and Dwellings

O. Axelson

Department of Occupational Medicine, University Hospital, 581 85 Linköping, Sweden

Since the late 1970s, radon in the human environment has become a major health interest with regard to risk of cancer. Radon is an inert gas emanating from the ground and stony building materials, and increased concentrations typically occur in underground mines but quite often also in buildings. This element, more precisely radon-222, originates from the decay of uranium through radium, and the further decay of radon leads to a series of radioactive isotopes of polonium, bismuth, and lead. The first four of these isotopes are referred to as short-lived radon progeny (or radon daughters) and have half-lives from less than a millisecond up to almost 27 min. There is also a decay chain from thorium through radon-220, or thoron, but the elements in this series are usually of less hygienic concern.

Like radon-222 itself, also the decay products polonium-218 and polonium-214 emit alpha-particles. When radon progeny is inhaled and deposited in the respiratory tract, the result is an alpha-irradiation of the bronchial epithelium from these isotopes, whereas the contribution from the radon gas is marginal. The alpha-particles travel less than 100 μm into the tissue, but their high energy causes an intense local ionization and a risk for subsequent cancer development. There is also beta- and gamma-radiation from some of the decay products of radon, but with much lower energy content than the alpha-radiation and therefore considered relatively unimportant.

Lung cancer is the only type of malignancy that has been clearly associated with exposure to radon and radon progeny and was first seen among miners. The potential health hazard for the general population of indoor exposure levels has not yet been well established, but it is of some interest in this context that already long ago, some circumstances in the epidemiology of lung cancer suggested an etiological influence from (an)other widespread factor(s) than smoking. This may even be the reason why critical comments have been made from time to time with regard to the causality of smoking and lung cancer (Passey 1962; Burch 1978, 1982). For example, the urban-rural difference in lung cancer rates may be recalled, as well as the influence of immigration on lung cancer morbidity, along with the varying lung cancer rates over the world, also when smoking is allowed for (Dean 1961, 1979; Burch 1978). An inverse relation of lung cancer and inhalation of cigarette smoke has been reported

(Fisher 1959; Higenbottam et al. 1982) and is a puzzling phenomenon for which different explanations might be offered (Wald et al. 1983; Axelson 1984). Furthermore, it has been a matter of some consideration why bronchitis but not lung cancer has shown the better correlation with air pollution (WHO 1972).

The relatively recent recognition of a widespread exposure to indoor radon and its decay products may open a new perspective and explain some of the less clear phenomena noted in lung cancer epidemiology, and perhaps also provide a possibility for prevention in addition to decreasing smoking. With a starting point in mining, the intention is here to elucidate the relation of lung cancer to radon and its decay products, particularly with regard to indoor exposure. It is unavoidable, however, that an evaluation in this respect will suffer from the scanty data on the risk of radon in homes as available at this time. A related aspect that is brought up in this review concerns the methodologic difficulties in studies of lung cancer and indoor radon progeny exposure.

Mining and Lung Cancer from Past to Present

An excess of lung cancer in miners was first reported in 1879 from Schneeberg in what is now the German Democratic Republic (GDR) (Härting and Hesse 1879), and in the beginning of this centuary also from Joachimsthal in Czechoslovakia (Arnstein 1913). Long before, however, and already in the sixteenth centuary, both Paracelsus and Agricola had described a high mortality from pulmonary disorders among miners, presumably predominated by lung cancer. In 1924 it was first suggested that the radioactivity found in the mine atmosphere could be responsible for this disorder (Ludewig and Lorenser 1924). This view was not generally accepted, however, and, for example, as late as in 1944, it was argued that a genetic susceptibility of the miners could be responsible for their lung cancer (Lorenz 1944). It was not until the 1950s and 1960s, that the etiological role of radon and its decay products was more fully understood and agreed upon.

An important step towards risk assessment for miners was taken in the 1950s, when the working level (WL) concept was introduced as a measure of the level of exposure to radon progeny (Holaday 1955). One working level is any combination of short-lived radon progeny in 1 l of air that will ultimately release 1.3×10^5 MeV of alpha energy by decay through polonium-214. This amount of radon progeny may also be taken as equivalent to 3700 Bq/m^3 EER (equilibrium equivalent radon; ICRP 1976) or 2.08×10^{-5} J/m^3. The accumulated exposure to radiation is expressed in terms of working level months (WLM), with the month in this context corresponding to 170 h exposure. The corresponding SI unit is the joule-hour per cubic meter, and 1 WLM is equal to 3.6×10^{-3} J-h/m^3 and may also be taken as 72 Bq-years/m^3.

Occupational exposure levels have been high in the past, especially in uranium mines. The extreme exposure situation may be well illustrated by mentioning the need for an exposure category of 3720 WLM and over in one study of uranium miners (Lundin et al. 1971). The radon progeny concentrations in many nonuranium mines have been about 1 WL or more. For example, hematite mines in West Cumberland, Great Britain, used to have exposure levels of 0.15–3.2 WL (Boyd et al. 1970). The cumulated annual exposure of French miners has been reported as 2.5–4.3 WLM during the late 1950s and 1960s but decreased to 1.6–3.2 WLM during the following decade (Tirmarche et al. 1985).

The introduction of 4 WLM per year as cumulative exposure limit in many countries during the 1970s has considerably improved the conditions in many mines. For example, the exposure levels in Swedish mines are now about 0.1 WL or below in contrast to commonly occurring levels of 0.5 to 1 WL or more around 1970. However, still in 1986, the US Mine Safety and Health Administration reported 19 out of 254 operating nonuranium mines to have exposure levels at 0.3 WL or more (NIOSH 1987). Such levels would lead to cumulated exposures close to or above the limit of 4 WLM per year.

Many mining populations with exposure to radon and decay products have been studied since the 1960s by the cohort as well as the case-control technique, e.g., uranium miners in the US, Canada, Czechoslovakia and France (Lundin et al. 1971; Sevc et al. 1976; Kunz et al. 1978; Waxweiler et al. 1981; Chovil and Chir 1981; Muller et al. 1985; Tirmarche et al. 1985), iron and other metal miners in the US, UK, China, France, and Sweden (Wagoner et al. 1963; Boyd et al. 1970; Axelson and Rehn 1971; Jörgensen 1973; Axelson and Sundell 1978; Fox et al. 1981; Damber and Larsson 1982; Edling and Axelson 1983; Wang et al. 1984; Radford and Renard 1984), and also fluorspar miners in Canada (deVilliers and Windish 1964; Morrison et al. 1985). All these exposed populations show a consistently increased risk of lung cancer, even if the overall risk ratios in the various studies have ranged from about 1.5 to 15. Tables 1 and 2 give some examples of these studies and the results obtained. Other cancer forms than lung cancer have not been clearly related to radon progeny exposure in mines, although a few studies have shown a tendency towards an excess of stomach cancer (BEIR IV 1988).

In contrast, miners with a very low exposure to radon and decay products have had little or no excess of lung cancer, i.e., in coal (IARC 1987) and potash mining (Waxweiler et al. 1973) and also in iron mining (Lawler et al. 1985). It seems quite convincing, therefore, that the radioactivity rather than other factors in the mine atmosphere is mainly responsible for the lung cancer risk, even if some other agents may be thought of as possibly contributing, e.g., diesel fumes and carcinogenic trace metals in the dust, especially arsenic when present. Asbestiform fibers have occurred in some Swedish mines at least, although they are less likely to have played any substantial role for lung cancer in this context (Edling 1982). It has also become clear in recent years that silica dust exposure may be associated with a lung cancer risk (IARC 1987), and some contribution in this respect to miners' lung cancer cannot be ruled out.

Table 1. Summary of some cohort studies of lung cancer mortality in underground mine workers exposed to radon progeny. (Modified from NIOSH 1987)

Type of mine (location)	Mean life-time exposure or concentration	Person-years	Lung cancer deaths			Reference
			Observed	Expected	SMR	
Metal (US)	0.05–0.40 WL	23 862	47	16.1	292	Wagoner et al. (1963)
Uranium (US)	821 WLM	62 556	185	38.4	482	Waxweiler et al. (1981) Lundin et al. (1971)
Uranium (Czechoslovakia)	289 WLM	56 955	211	42.7	496	Placek et al. (1983); Kunz et al. (1978)
Tin (United Kingdom)	1.2–3.4 WL	27 631	28	13.27	211	Fox et al. (1981)
Iron (Sweden)	0.5 WL	10 230	28	6.79	412	Jörgensen (1984)
Iron (Sweden)	81.4 WLM	24 083	50	12.8	390	Radford and Renard (1984)
Fluorspar (Canada)	Up to 2040 WLM	37 730	104	24.38	427	Morrison et al. (1985)
Uranium (Canada)	40–90 WLM	202 795	82	56.9	144	Muller et al. (1985)
Uranium (Canada)	17 WLM	118 341	65	34.24	190	Howe et al. (1986)

SMR, standardized mortality ratio.

Table 2. Summary of some case-control studies of lung cancer mortality in underground mine workers exposed to radon progeny

Type of mine (location)	Estimated concentration or exposure	Cases/ controls (n)	Exposed cases (n)	Rate ratio for lung cancer deaths	Reference
Zinc-lead (Sweden)	1 WL	29/174	21	16.4	Axelson and Sundell (1978)
Iron (Sweden)	0.1–2.0 WL	604/(467 × 2 + 137)	20	7.3	Damber and Larsson (1982)
Iron (Sweden)	0.3 to 1.0 WL	38/403	33	11.5	Edling and Axelson (1983)
Uranium (US)	Lifetime exposure: 30 to 2698 WLM	32/64	23	Infinite	Samet et al. (1984)

Indoor Radon as an Emerging Health Hazard

Indoor radon depends on both building material and ground conditions. The leakage of radon from the ground is a somewhat irregular phenomenon and may vary locally within a few meters due to cracks and porosity of the ground. When very high indoor concentrations occur, leakage from the ground is usually more important than the emanation from the building materials of a house (Åkerblom and Wilson 1982). Temperature and wind conditions, air pressure, but also behavioral factors influence ventilation, which plays a major role for the concentrations that may build up in a room. The introduction of central heating as reducing the thermal ventilation in comparison to houses with fireplaces, as well as the more recent efforts to improve insulation and preserve energy, are likely to have caused quite considerable increases of indoor radon concentrations since the beginning of this century (Dickson 1978; Stranden et al. 1979; McGregor et al. 1980).

The first measurements of indoor radon were undertaken in Sweden already in the 1950s (Hultqvist 1956), but seem to have attracted little interest from the health point of view. The levels found at that time were in the range of 20–69 Bq/m^3 (0.005–0.019 WL). More recent measurements in Swedish homes have revealed higher levels, i.e., 122 Bq/m^3 (0.033 WL) as an average in detached houses and 85 Bq/m^3 (0.023 WL) in apartments, but there are such great variations as from 11–3300 Bq/m^3 (0.003–0.892 WL) (Swedjemark et al. 1987). The differences between the early and the more recently measured concentrations should probably be interpreted as suggesting a general increase in the levels over time.

Average or median concentrations of indoor radon in the range of 40–100 Bq/m^3 have been reported from many countries, e.g., USA (Nero et al. 1986), Norway (Stranden 1987), Finland (Castren et al. 1987), Federal Republic of Germany (Schmier and Wick 1985). High levels, like 2000 or 3000 Bq/m^3, may occur in many houses, and this is about double the level tolerated in mines in most countries (about 1100 Bq/m^3 or 0.3 WL). The considerable variation in concentrations between houses and over time clearly indicates the potential difficulties involved in assessing individual exposures for epidemiologic studies; this will be further discussed.

Design Issues in Studies of Exposure to Indoor Radon Progeny

Since about 1979, a number of epidemiologic studies have been undertaken to evaluate the possible role of indoor radon for the lung cancer risk of the general population. These studies have often been of the case-control type, but several correlation studies have also been published regarding the occurrence of lung cancer in various countries or regions in relation to quite crude estimates of radon in homes.

A major problem in epidemiologic studies is always to obtain proper exposure information and the studying of radon progeny exposure in the general environment and lung cancer is no exception; indeed, the problem is even greater than in many other studies, since the individual has no perception of exposure and usually has lived in many houses with varying exposure levels. Some people spend most of their indoor time at home, whereas others prefer to more often be out in the open air or have indoor activities in various other houses with different radon concentrations. Only the exposure in the home environment would be reasonably easy to estimate in retrospect; however, great uncertainties affect any exposure assessment. It is also obvious that even quite extensive measurements in a number of subsequently used homes of an individual would not permit any particularly good estimate of his or her cumulated exposure over many decades. Nevertheless, a combination of measurements and judgements with regard to pertinent characteristics of a house might be assumed to give a usable estimate of radon progeny exposure.

By restricting a study population to be rural, the precision in the assessment of individual exposure may improve. The reason for this is that the subjects involved, especially the women, are more likely to have spent most indoor time in their homes, whereas the situation in this respect may be quite different for an urban population. Furthermore, a rural population tends to be very stable and many individuals were even born in the same house where they died.

In view of such considerations, some of the first studies were restricted to rural populations (Axelson et al. 1979; Edling et al. 1984). The building material of the house where a subject had lived just prior to death was considered in terms of wooden versus stone as indicative of indoor radon levels according to the early measurements by Hultqvist (1956). However, a mixed category was used when the house had some other, less distinct character. The existence of a basement was also taken into account as possibly increasing the indoor radon levels.

Some further refinement in estimating exposure through indirect methods was applied in the second of these studies, i.e., from the island of Oeland in the Baltic (Edling et al. 1984). This island has quite specific geological features, i.e., along the west coast there is an alum shale strip leaking radon, which could be taken into account as likely to contribute to indoor radon. The population density is high in this very clearly defined zone, which is only a few hundred meters in breadth, whereas the rest of the island consists of lime and sandstone with a low radon emanation. Geophysical maps were also available indicating the increased background radiation of the alum shale zone. Cellulose nitrate film measurements of indoor radon progeny concentrations were also undertaken and found to agree relatively well with the exposure categories based on various characteristics of the houses and their locations as likely to have determined indoor radon concentrations. Furthermore, the study of the Oeland population only included individuals who had lived in the same house for 30 years or more. This restriction strongly reduced the number of individuals eligible for the study, but was likely to improve the accuracy of the exposure, i.e., with regard to the specific exposure category ascribed to each individual.

Other investigators in the field have applied similar classifications of assumed exposure, i.e., with regard to type of house construction and building material, as, for example, in a study from Maryland (Simpson and Comstock 1983). Some very distinct assumptions were made in one study, as the exposure was estimated in terms of $kBq/m^3 \times$ months (Pershagen et al. 1984). Considering all the uncertainties involved in the exposure assessment in this context, a more crude classification based on building material in the walls, only distinguishing between wood and other (stony) materials (Damber and Larsson 1986), might perhaps be as efficient. This approach has also been used as an alternative assessment of exposure in a recent study (Axelson et al. 1988).

In still another study of an urban population in the Stockholm area, it was required for the classification of an individual as more exposed that she (only women were included in the study) had lived either in a detached house or at the bottom floor of a multifamily house, i.e., under circumstances implying exposure to relatively higher radon concentrations (Svensson et al. 1987). Measurements were made in 10% of the houses and, in addition, there was already some further information available regarding radon emanation from the ground in certain sectors of the geographical area involved. Finally, there are a few studies, in which the exposure has been entirely based on direct measurements (Lanes et al. 1982; Lanes 1983).

In correlation studies, general information about background radiation and data on radon in water etc. have been utilized as the exposure variable (Edling et al. 1982; Bean et al. 1982; Hess et al. 1983; Hofmann et al. 1985; Dousset and

Jammet 1985; Forastiere et al. 1985). Other cancers than lung cancer have also been considered in some of these studies.

Results in Studies of Exposure to Indoor Radon Progeny

All of the clear-cut case-control studies available so far have shown some degree of increased lung cancer risk in relation to assumed elevated levels of indoor radon progeny. On the average, the risk ratios have been around 2, but higher for particular subgroups (Table 3). One of the studies considered oat-cell and other anaplastic lung cancers in women only (Svensson et al. 1987). Another study reported a relative predominance of squamous and small cell carcinomas among those who had lived in nonwooden houses, i.e., under assumed elevated exposure to radon progeny indoors (Damber and Larsson 1986).

Simpson and Comstock (1983) followed a mixed rural-urban population of 39 636 individuals in Maryland, USA, for the period 1963–1975 with regard to lung cancer among people who had lived in houses of different constructions and building materials. The study included 298 lung cancer cases. No clear effect was seen, but somewhat higher lung cancer rates were associated with concrete in the walls and with a construction on a concrete slab, especially for those

Table 3. Results in studies of lung cancer and exposure to indoor radon and radon daughters (case-control studies)

Author and year	Cases to controls (*n*)	Rate ratio(s)	Remarks (CI)
Axelson et al. (1979)	37/178	1.8	CI 90, 0.99–3.2
Edling et al. (1984)	23/202	Up to 4.3	CI 90, 1.7–10.6
Pershagen et al. (1984)	Two sets of 30/30	–	Significantly higher exposure for smoking cases; no clear difference vs controls for the nonsmokers
Damber and Larson (1986)	604/(467 × 2 + 137)	Up to 2.0	CI 95, 1.0–4.1 (for more than 20 years in nonwooden houses)
Svensson et al. (1987)	292/584	2.2	CI 95, 1.2–4.0, women with oat-cell carcinoma
Lees et al. (1987)	27/49	Up to 11.9	Risk of 11.9 corresponding to 10 WLM of exposure in regression model
Lanes et al. (1982)	50/50	2.1	Published abstract only

CI, confidence interval.

having lived in such houses for 15 years or more. These particular relationships may be best explained as an effect of radon progeny exposure.

Several of the correlation studies indicate a more or less clear relationship between the occurrence of lung cancer and some indirect measure of potential radon emission from the ground. For example, geological features such as phosphate deposits, that had been worked (Fleischer 1981), or volcanic versus sedimentary structures (Forastiere et al. 1985), have been utilized to create a contrast in exposure. The occurrence of a type of granite with increased radioactivity has provided another opportunity for a study on a county basis, contrasting the lung cancer rates of the populations within and without the area with the particular granite (Archer 1987). Estimated average background radiation levels per county have also been utilized as a surrogate for potential indoor radon (Edling et al. 1982). Some other of these somewhat crude, but more or less positive studies, have been based on measurements of Ra-226 in water (Bean et al. 1982) or investigated levels of radon in water and indoor air (Hess et al. 1983).

In some of these studies, a correlation has been obtained also for other cancers than lung cancer, e.g., for pancreatic cancer and male leukemia (Edling et al. 1982), bladder and breast cancer (Bean et al. 1982), and for reproductive cancer in males as well as for all cancers taken together (Hess et al. 1983). A high mortality rate from stomach cancer has been reported from New Mexico in an area with uranium deposits (Wilkinson 1985). This excess of cancers other than lung cancer might be an effect of other decay products from uranium, than the inhaled short-lived radon progeny, say radium in drinking water. It is not immediately clear, however, if this increased cancer mortality at all can be attributed to radioactivity.

Some correlation studies have also come out negative with regard to lung cancer, e.g., from Canada (Létourneau et al. 1983), China (Hofmann et al. 1985), and France (Dousset and Jammet 1985). The latter study, undertaken in an area with higher assumed indoor radon levels, showed some excess of digestive tract cancers.

Based on this short review of the literature, it may be concluded, that in most of the studies published so far, there has appeared some increase in the risk of lung cancer in relation to the estimates used for exposure to elevated indoor levels of radon progeny. There might be indirect relations with some other cancers as well, i.e., increased levels of radon tend to be associated with the occurrence of other radioactive materials, which may or may not explain some of the observations made.

Review of Some Recent Studies

In view of the present interest for the potential lung cancer hazard from indoor radon, it is not surprising that studies in this respect has started in several countries or are being planned, e.g., in the USA, UK, Belgium and elsewhere in

Europe. For example, a rather large Swedish study may be mentioned as in progress, involving 1500 lung cancer cases and two sets of controls, 1500 in each. This study is supposed to take about 5 years to finish, and some results may be expected in 1992.

The results from two new Swedish studies may deserve a more detailed review. One of these studies (Svensson et al. 1988) is based on 210 incident female lung cancer cases and two control groups, i.e., one series involving 209 matched population controls and the other 191 hospital controls. Exposure to indoor radon progeny was assessed by means of estimations and also measurements in 10.9% of the dwellings held for more than 2 years by the subjects; in addition the dwellings were classified with regard to whether or not there was a ground contact that likely would have increased indoor radon. Risk ratios of 1.8 and 1.7 were obtained for the medium and high categories of cumulated exposure, respectively, with the strongest effect for small cell carcinoma and lowest for adenocarcinoma. Squamous and small cell carcinomas taken together resulted in risk ratios of 2.3 and 3.1 in the respective exposure categories. Furthermore, these risks operated primarily among the smokers, and it might be added that smoking, as controlled in the study, was negatively associated with estimated radon progeny exposure.

The other of the two new Swedish studies (Axelson et al. 1988) is very similar to the earlier one from the island of Oeland (Edling et al. 1984). Hence, this study was again confined to an area with alum shale deposits in central south Sweden, because the idea was to obtain an exposure contrast between the houses due to local differences in radon emanation from the ground. Also building material and character of the houses were taken into account for the assessment of exposure. As a matter of fact it was possible to apply exactly the same criteria for classification of exposure as was used in the study from Oeland. This new study is larger, however, encompassing 177 cases and 673 referents. Measurements were possible in 143 of the case houses, whereas economic constraints reduced the number of measured referent houses relatively more, i.e., to 251. Again all subjects were required to have lived at the same, last address for at least 30 years.

The current levels of indoor radon progeny corresponding to the exposure categories chosen turned out to be 112 (0.030 WL), 97 (0.026 WL), and 57 Bq/m^3 EER (0.015 WL), respectively, in those houses that were measured with alpha-sensitive film. With regard to alternative, dichotomized categories based on wall materials only, measured values varied from 151 Bq/m^3 EER (0.041 WL) for light weight alum shale concrete or mixed materials to 87 Bq/m^3 EER (0.024 WL) for wood, brick, and other stony material, the latter apparently without any particularly high radioactivity.

The result of the study has relatively well reproduced the findings from the earlier studies of our group (Axelson et al. 1979; Edling et al. 1984; the method sections of these papers also give the references for the various epidemiologic concepts used below). Hence, the risk ratios over the exposure categories were 1.0, 1.5, and 1.8, respectively. However, by considering age, sex, smoking habits, and urban-rural distribution by stratification, it appeared that nonsmokers, passive smokers, and occasional smokers in rural areas showed an increasing risk with higher category of assumed exposure, whereas there was no such definite pattern for the smokers, nor in the urban population irrespective of smoking habits. The same findings also appeared for the subset of cases and controls for whom there were measurements of indoor radon daughter levels. It might be added, though, that only cases and no controls appeared among the smokers in the highest exposure category based on the measurements. With regard to wall materials in the homes, the risk ratio was 2.0 (and the 90% confidence interval, CI 90 was 1.1–3.7) for residents in the houses with high versus low radon daughter levels; this analysis involved both the rural and urban population sector.

Considering passive and occasional smokers together (the latter likely to be particularly tolerant to environmental tobacco smoke), and aggregating both rural and urban areas, the crude risk ratios were 1.0, 2.1, and 2.3 with regard to the exposure categories. By stratification on age, sex, and urban-rural distribution, the corresponding Mantel-Haenszel risk ratios were 1.0, 1.9 (CI 90, 0.78–4.5) and 2.9 (CI 90, 1.2–6.6), respectively. Passive smoking only, without any consideration of radon progeny exposure, resulted in a crude risk ratio of 1.2 with a corresponding Mantel-Haenszel risk ratio of 0.9 after stratification as above. This means that there was no clear effect in these data with regard to passive smoking only.

The interpretation of this study might be that some further support has been obtained for the proposition that exposure to indoor radon progeny may play a relatively important role for lung cancer. This view seems reasonable in spite of the internally somewhat inconsistent findings for the rural and urban population sector. It is more relevant namely, if the rural population appears to be affected by lung cancer in relation to degree of assumed exposure, because rural people are apt to spend most indoor time at home rather than in other buildings. The habits in urban areas are obviously quite different in this respect. There are also many occupational factors operating in an urban population and general air pollution in densely populated areas may also play some role in obscuring an effect of indoor radon progeny exposure. Furthermore, the study had no subdivision of the smokers into consumption categories, which may imply a somewhat poor control of confounding, should it be negative and masking an effect. Some further support for a lung cancer risk from indoor exposure to radon progeny is obtained from the fact that an increased risk appeared with regard to certain wall materials as rather well correlating with high radon progeny concentrations in the measurements.

On the Combined Effect of Smoking and Exposure to Radon Progeny

Most of the studies of miners suggest a multiplicative interaction or synergism between smoking and radon progeny exposure, but a few studies have also suggested a merely additive relationship or even less than an additive effect. This discrepancy between various studies may seem disturbing, but conceptually there is not necessarily any definite inconsistency. Instead, the explanation might be that there is an influence of smoking on mucous secretion and, therefore, also on the thickness of the mucous sheath, which in turn would determine the number of alpha-particles able to penetrate to the basal cells of the epithelium from which cancer may develop.

Increased mucous secretion in the respiratory tract may occur especially among smokers, when exposed to dusty ambient air as occurred in some older mines, where a merely additive or subadditive interaction has been observed with regard to smoking, radon progeny exposure, and lung cancer (Axelson and Sundell 1978; Dahlgren 1979; Edling 1982). It may be recalled in this context, that a considerably increased prevalence of bronchitis has been reported in smoking miners (Sluis-Cremer et al. 1967; Jörgensen and Swensson 1970), but the criteria used for the diagnosis of this disorder may not clearly distinguish a simple mucous hypersecretion from true bronchitis. It is noteworthy also, that an increase in thickness of the mucous layer of only about 10 μm would decrease the dose to the epithelium by the order of some 50% (Altshuler et al. 1964; Walsh 1970). However, with regard to cancer development, there is also likely to be a synergism between chemicals in tobacco smoke and the actual dose of radiation to the epithelium. This is indicated by the more or less multiplicative interaction found in many of the studies of miners. Evidence in this direction has also been obtained from sputum cytology of uranium miners (Band et al. 1980).

The somewhat complex view given here on the interaction of smoking and radon progeny exposure seems to be quite well supported by animal experiments. For example, it has been reported that smoking dogs were less affected by respiratory cancer than nonsmoking dogs, when both groups were exposed to uranium ore dust and radon progeny (Cross et al. 1982). However, there are also experiments in rodents indicating that radon progeny exposure followed by exposure to cigarette smoke stimulated tumour development, whereas the reverse combination did not (Chameaud et al. 1985). A double role of smoking as both influencing the mucous secretion and subsequently the dose obtained, as well as the cancer process itself, seems therefore plausible but might also lead to almost any overall epidemiologic result, i.e., from a multiplicative to an even less than additive effect dependent on the particular circumstances under which exposure occurs.

Also for exposure to indoor radon progeny and smoking, there seems to be a more or less multiplicative effect, although only a few studies provide data in this respect. Especially in rural areas this pattern of interaction was seen (Edling et al. 1984; Edling and Axelson 1987) and has appeared also for passive and occasional smokers (Axelson et al. 1988). It has to be pointed out, however, that there are also some inconsistencies between the various studies, especially with regard to smokers in urban areas (Svensson et al. 1987, 1988; Axelson et al. 1988). There may be several reasons for these inconsistencies, e.g., simply the instability of the estimates due to the relatively small numbers involved in the studies as further underscored by the different effects indicated for the various histological types of lung cancer (Svensson et al. 1988). Similarly as in studies of miners (Archer et al. 1974; Horacek et al. 1977), small cell carcinomas showed the strongest ássociation with indoor exposure to radon progeny. This relationship has been indicated also in the earlier studies (Damber and Larsson 1986; Svensson et al. 1987).

A further aspect on the interaction of smoking and radon progeny exposure may be brought up in this context, namely the tendency of radon progeny to attach to environmental tobacco smoke. This phenomenon increases the airborne radioactivity in the presence of tobacco smoke, i.e., there is less plating out of radon progeny on walls, furniture, and other surfaces in a room (Bergman et al. 1986). As a consequence, however, the fraction of unattached progeny tends to be reduced. The biological net effect of this increased radioactivity of the smoke-polluted air and the reduction of unattached progeny is not clear. Usually, the unattached fraction has been considered as more important than the attached fraction for the radiation dose to the epithelium, but a large part of the unattached progeny tends to be deposited rather high up in the respiratory tract, at least by nose breathing. In this region, however, the epithelium is thick enough to hinder penetration of the alpha-particles to the basal cells, from which cancer may develop (Walsh 1970). In contrast, the smoke-attached progeny tend to be deposited further down the respiratory tract (George and Breslin 1969; Morken 1979), or in those bronchial regions where the cancers occur.

In the context of mining, the unattached fraction has usually been thought of as responsible for the greater part of the dose delivered to the bronchial epithelium, but the pattern of respiration would be characterized by more mouth breathing in heavy mining work than in sedentary situations in the home environment. Further work seems to be needed to permit a more elaborated view on this interaction of active as well as passive smoking and radon progeny exposure in various environments.

Comparing Risk Estimates in Miners and the General Population

Comprehensive reviews and estimations of the lung cancer risk from exposure to radon and its decay products have recently been elaborated (NIOSH 1987; BEIR IV 1988; IARC 1988) and involve reanalyses of previously presented data on miners along with new, quantitated risk assessments (NIOSH 1987; BEIR IV 1988). Comparisons with the risks noted in studies of general populations with indoor exposure to radon progeny would obviously be of great interest, but would involve great uncertainties due to sparsity of data.

NIOSH (1987) derived the risk estimation from uranium miners in the Colorado Plateau area as followed for many years (Lundin et al. 1971). The increase of the risk ratio was calculated to be 1.57 for a cumulated exposure of

30 WLM (above background) over a 30-year working life. The corresponding excess of lung cancer deaths per 1000 miners was estimated to 10 cases. For a cumulative exposure of 15 WLM, the risk ratio was estimated to be 1.31, and the expected excess of cases per 1000 miners was given as 4.9. In additive terms, exposures of 15 WLM as well as of 30 WLM and also some higher exposures, would result in an excess of about 0.33 cases per WLM and 1000 individuals over lifetime. Similarly, the BEIR IV (1988) report arrived at 0.35 cases per WLM and 1000 individuals over lifetime. The corresponding figures that can be derived from two of the house studies (Axelson et al. 1979; Edling et al. 1984) are in the range of 0.3–0.8 cases per WLM and 1000 individuals over lifetime (Edling and Axelson 1987). The small number of cases underlying these figures, makes the agreement with the risk estimate from the miners rather uncertain even if formally quite consistent.

As already indicated to some extent, NIOSH (1987) as well as BEIR IV (1988) advocated a multiplicative risk model for the lung cancer effect of radon progeny exposure, whereas earlier risk assessments usually have presumed additivity. A multiplicative model implies synergistic effects with other causes of lung cancer as influencing the background rate of this disease, notably smoking, but also with earlier exposure to radon progeny, both occupational and background in character.

The multiplicative risk model makes it somewhat simpler to more directly involve case-control data from studies of the general population in comparisons with cohort studies of miners. This may be looked upon as a simplification that, if tenable, probably will turn out to be valuable, since it is likely that most studies of radon progeny exposure in general populations also in the future will be of a case-control design, particularly for reasons of costs. Data from one of the house studies (Axelson et al. 1988) may immediately be used in this model for a crude comparison of predictable and observed risk ratios in relation to degree of exposure. Some approximations would be necessary, however, because of missing information or differences with regard to age stratification, etc.

The model given by the BEIR IV report may be presented as

$$R(a)/r(a) = 1 + 0.025\mu(a)(W + 0.5V)$$

where $R(a)$ is the lung cancer rate at age a among the exposed; $r(a)$ is the baseline rate (as in the 1980–1984 US population); $\mu(a)$ is 1.2 for ages less than 55 years, 1.0 for ages 55–64 years, and 0.4 for age 65 years or greater; W is the cumulated exposure in WLM from 5 to 15 years before age a; and V is the cumulative in WLM 15 years or more before age a. $R(a)/r(a)$ is then apparently the risk ratio at age a. It may be noted here that the model implies that relatively recent exposure would play a greater role for lung cancer development than usually assumed, i.e., exposure from the last 5 to 15 years has been given more weight than earlier exposure. This would imply that alpha-radiation operates as a late stage carcinogen, even if the animal experiments referred to also clearly suggest an early stage effect (Chameaud et al. 1985).

Considering the house study (Axelson et al. 1988), the μ-factor in the BEIR IV model may be taken as 0.8 as an average with regard to the relatively high ages for the lung cancer cases. Recent exposure, W, may be derived from an exposure level of 151 Bq/m^3 as a measured average for an elevated exposure category, as mentioned above. At the age of 60, say, and with some 80% indoor occupancy time, one obtains 25 WLM for the recent 15 years of exposure, W. Then, for the earlier period of life, i.e., until 45, V might be 50 WLM as accumulated (over three times as long a time) at those somewhat lower exposure levels, that are likely to have occurred in the past. Then, $(W+0.5V)$ would be 50 WLM and the rate ratio, $R(a)/r(a)$, is obtained as 2.0, or just as found in the study with regard to the exposure category with 151 Bq/m^3 as an average. Other similar comparisons are also possible and would show reasonable agreements as well.

Calculations of this kind may seem a bit primitive in view of the fact that the lung cancer risk of any reference population also has to be thought of as influenced by radon progeny exposure. However, this is something which is shared with the background population involved in the model for the miners and may therefore be thought of as allowed for.

Epilogue

In view of a number of recent epidemiologic studies it may be justified to believe that not only various miner groups but also large parts of the general population have a risk of lung cancer due to radon progeny exposure. Still there may be reasons to look critically at the comparisons made here between miners and general populations because of a possible influence from different other factors in mines and houses. Similarly, a critical view should be taken also with regard to the calculation of the increase in risk ratio in relation to exposure. A tentative conclusion could be that the lung cancer risk per amount of exposure to radon progeny very well can be quantitatively similar whether the radiation is obtained in mines or in homes. Further insights into the dose-response and time relationships of radon progeny exposure and the interaction with smoking in humans might be obtained from the studies under way on indoor exposure.

With regard to the lifetime risk of lung cancer in miners, one extra death per 1000 miners has been considered as possibly acceptable, but this would only permit an exposure of about 0.1 WLM per year (NIOSH 1987). However, already the average background exposure in the US was estimated to 0.2 WLM per year (and up to 0.4 WLM per year in the vicinity of radon emitting ore bodies), but the exposure even seems to be considerably higher for large population sectors in many other countries. This fact certainly illustrates the problem of prevention, not only in the context of mining, but especially with regard to indoor exposure to radon progeny.

References

Åkerblom G, Wilson C (1982) Radon – geological aspects of an environmental problem. Sveriges geologiska undersökning, Uppsala (Rapporter och meddelanden no 30)

Altshuler B, Nelson N, Kuschner M (1964) Estimation of lung tissue dose from the inhalation of radon and daughters. Health Phys 10: 1137–1161

Archer VE (1987) Association of lung cancer mortality with precambrian granite. Occup Environ Health 42: 87–91

Archer VE, Saccomanno G, Jones JH (1974) Frequency of different histologic types of bronchogenic carcinoma as related to radon exposure. Cancer 34: 2056–2060

Arnstein A (1913) Über den sogenannten "Schneeberger Lungenkrebs". Verh Dtsch Ges Pathol 16: 332–342

Axelson O (1984) Room for a role for radon in lung cancer causation? Med Hypotheses 13: 51–61

Axelson O, Rehn M (1971) Lung cancer in miners. Lancet ii: 706–707

Axelson O, Sundell L (1978) Mining, lung cancer and smoking, Scand J Work Environ Health 4: 46–52

Axelson O, Edling C, Kling H (1979) Lung cancer and residency – a case referent study on the possible impact of exposure to radon and its daughters in dwellings. Scand J Work Environ Health 5: 10–15

Axelson, O, Andersson K, Desai G, Fagerlund I, Jansson B, Karlsson C, Wingren G (1988) A case-referent study on lung cancer, indoor radon and active and passive smoking. Scand J Work Environ Health 14: 286–292

Band P, Feldstein M, Saccomanno G, Watson L, King G (1980) Potentiation of cigarette smoking and radiation. Evidence from a sputum cytology survey among uranium miners and controls. Cancer 45: 1273–1277

Bean JA, Isacson P, Hahne RMA, Kohler J (1982) Drinking water and cancer incidence in Iowa. Am J Epidemiol 116: 924–932

BEIR IV: Committee on the biological effects of ionizing radiations, US National Research Council (1988) Health risks of radon and other intervally deposited alpha-emitters. National Academy Press, Washington, D.C.

Bergman H, Edling C, Axelson O (1986) Indoor radon daughter concentrations and passive smoking. Environm Internat 12: 17–19

Boyd JP, Doll R, Faulds JS, Leiper J (1970) Cancer of the lung in iron ore (haematite) miners. Br J Ind Med 27: 97–105

Burch PRJ (1978) Smoking and lung cancer: the problem of inferring cause. J R Stat Soc 141(4): 437–477

Burch PRJ (1982) Cigarette smoking and lung cancer. Med Hypotheses 9: 293–306

Castren O, Mäkeläinen I, Winqvist K, Voutilainen A (1987) Indoor radon measurements in Finland: a status report. In: Hopke PK (ed) Radon and its decay products – occurrence, properties and health effects. American Chemical Society, Washington DC, pp 97–103

Chemeaud J, Masse R, Morin M, Lafuma J (1985) Lung cancer induction by radon daughters in rats; present state of the date in low dose exposures. In: Stocker (ed) Proceedings of the International Conference on Occupational Radiation Safety in Mining. Canadian Nuclear Association, Toronto, pp 350–353

Chovil A, Chir B (1981) The epidemiology of primary lung cancer in uranium miners in Ontario. J Occup Med 23: 417–421

Cross FT, Palmer RF, Filipy RE, Dagle GE, Stuart BO (1982) Carcinogenic effects of radon daughters, uranium ore dust and cigarette smoke in beagle dogs. Health Phys 42: 33–52

Dahlgren E (1979) Lungcancer, cardiovascular disease and smoking in a group of miners. Translation of: Lungcancer, hjärt-kärlsjukdom och rökning hos en grupp gruvarbetare. Läkartidningen 76: 4811–4814

Damber L, Larsson LG (1982) Combined effects of mining and smoking in the causation of lung cancer. A case-control study. Acta Radiol Oncol 21: 305–315

Damber L, Larsson LG (1986) Lung cancer in males and type of dwelling. An epidemiological pilot study. In: Damber L (ed) Lung cancer in males. An epidemiological study in northern Sweden with special regard to smoking and occupation. Thesis University of Umeå, Umeå (New series no 167)

Dean G (1961) Lung cancer among white South Africans. Br Med J 2: 1599–1605

Dean G (1979) The effects of air pollution and smoking on health in England, South Africa and Ireland. J Ir Med Assoc 72: 284–289

de Villiers AJ, Windish JP (1964) Lung cancer in a fluorspar mining community. I. Radiation, dust and mortality experience. Br J Ind Med 21: 94–109

Dickson D (1978) Home insulation may increase radiation hazard. Nature 276: 431

Dousset M, Jammet H (1985) Comparaison de la mortalité par cancer dans le Limousin et le Poitou-Charentes. Radioprotection GEDIM 20: 61–67

Edling C (1982) Lung cancer and smoking in a group of iron ore miners. Am J Ind Med 3: 191–199

Edling C, Axelson O (1983) Quantitative aspects of radon daughter exposure and lung cancer in underground miners. Br J Ind Med 40: 182–187

Edling C, Axelson O (1987) Radon daughter exposure, smoking and lung cancer. Clin Ecology 5 (2): 59–64

Edling C, Comba P, Axelson O, Flodin U (1982) Effects of low-dose radiation – a correlation study. Scand J Work Environ Health 8 [Suppl 1]: 59–64

Edling C, Kling H, Axelson O (1984) Radon in homes – a possible cause of lung cancer. Scand J Work Environ Health 10: 25–34

Fisher RA (1959) Smoking. The cancer controversy: some attempts to assess the evidence. Oliver and Boyd, Edinburgh

Fleischer RL (1981) A possible association between lung cancer and phosphate mining and processing. Health Phys 41: 171–175

Forastiere F, Valesini S, Arca M, Magliola ME, Michelozzi P, Tasco C (1985) Lung cancer and natural radiation in an Italian province. Sci Total Environ 45: 519–526

Fox AJ, Goldblatt P, Kinlen LJ (1981) A study of the mortality of Cornish tin miners. Br J Ind Med 38: 378

George AC, Breslin AJ (1969) Deposition of radon daughters in humans exposed to uranium mine atmospheres. Health Phys 17: 115–124

Härting FH, Hesse W (1879) Der Lungenkrebs, die Bergkrankheit in den Schneeberger Gruben. Vierteljahrsschrift für gerichtliche Medizin und öffentliches Gesundheitswesen 30: 296–309, 31: 102–132, 31: 313–337

Hess CT, Weiffenbach CV, Norton SA (1983) Environmental radon and cancer correlations in Maine. Health Phys 45: 339–348

Higenbottam T, Shipley MJ, Rose G (1982) Cigarettes, lung cancer, and coronary heart disease: the effects of inhalation and tar yield. J Epidemiol Community Health 36: 113–117

Hofmann W, Katz R, Zhang C (1985) Lung cancer incidence in a Chinese high background area-epidemiological results and theoretical interpretation. Sci Total Environ 45: 527–534

Holaday DA (1955) Digest of the proceedings of the 7-state conference on health hazards in uranium mining. Arch Ind Health 12: 465–467

Horácek J, Placek V, Sevc J (1977) Histologic types of bronchogenic cancer in relation to different conditions of radiation exposure. Cancer 34: 832–835

Howe GR, Nair RC, Newcombe HB, Miller AB, Frost SE, Abbatt JD (1986) Lung cancer mortality (1950–1980) in relation to radon daughter in a cohort of workers at the Eldorado Beaverlodge uranium mine. JNCI 77(2): 357–362

Hultqvist B (1956) Studies on naturally occurring ionizing radiations with special reference to radiation dose in Swedish houses of various types. Almqvist and Wiksell, Stockholm (Kungl Svenska vetenskapsakademiens handlingar, 4th ser, vol 6, no 3)

IARC (1987) Monographs on the evaluation of carcinogenic risks to humans, suppl 7. International Agency for Research on Cancer, Lyon

IARC (1988) Monographs on the evaluation of carcinogenic risks to humans. Man-made mineral fibres and radon Vol. 43 International Agency for Research on Cancer, Lyon

ICRP: International Commission on Radiological Protection (1976) Radiation protection in uranium and other mines. Pergamon, Oxford (ICRP publ no 24)

Jörgensen HS (1973) A stuty of mortality from lung cancer among miners in Kiruna 1950–1970. Work Environ Health 10: 126–133

Jörgenesen HS (1984) Lung cancer among underground workers in the iron ore mine of Kiruna based on thirty years of observation. Ann Acad Med Singapore 13: 371–377

Jörgensen H, Swensson A (1970) Investigation of workers in a mine with diesel drift, especially regarding lung function, respiratory symptoms and smoking habits. Translation of: Undersökning av arbetare i gruva med dieseldrift, särskilt med hänsyn till lungfunktion, luftvägssymtom och rökvanor. Arbetarskyddsverket, Stockholm (AI rapport no 16) (English summary)

Kunz E, Sevc J, Placek V (1978) Lung cancer in uranium miners. Health Phys 35: 579–580

Lanes SF (1983) Lung cancer and environmental radon exposure: a case-control study. Dissertation Abstr Int 43: 2787B–2788B

Lanes SF, Talbott E, Radford E (1982) Lung cancer and environmental radon. Am J Epidemiol 116: 565

Lawler AB, Mandel JS, Schuman LM, Lubin JH (1985) A retrospective cohort mortality study of iron ore (hemitite) miners in Minnesota. J Occup Med 27: 507–517

Lees REM, Steele R, Robert JH (1987) A case-control study of lung cancer relative to domestic radon exposure. Int J Epidemiol 16: 7–12

Letourneau EG, Mao Y, McGregor RG, Semenciw R, Smith MH, Wigle DT (1983) Lung cancer mortality and indoor radon concentrations in 18 Canadian cities. In: Proceedings of the sixteenth midyear topical meeting of the Health Physics Society on Epidemiology applied to health physics, Albuquerque, 9–13 Jan 1983. Health Physics Society, Ottawa, pp 470–483

Lorenz E (1944) Radioactivity and lung cancer: a critical review of lung cancer in the miners of Schneeberg and Joachimsthal. J NCI 5: 1–15

Ludewig P, Lorenser E (1924) Untersuchung der Grubenluft in den Schneeberger Gruben auf den Gehalt und Radiumemanation. Strahlenterapie 17: 428–435

Lundin FE Jr, Wagoner JK, Archer VE (1971) Radon daughter exposure and respiratory cancer. Quantitative and temporal aspects. US Department of Health, Education, and Welfare. Public Health Service, Springfield Va (NIOSH-NIEHS Joint monograph no 1)

McGregor RG, Vasudev P, Létourneau EG, McCullough RS, Prantl FA, Taniguchi H (1980) Background concentrations of radon and radon daughters in Canadian homes. Health Phys 39: 285–289

Morken DA (1979) The biological and health effects of radon: a review. In: Proceedings of a roundtable discussion of radon in buildings, Gaithersburg Md. National Bureau of Standards, Washington DC, pp 21–26 (National Bureau of Standards Special Publ no 581)

Morrison HI, Semenicw RM, Mao Y, Corkill DA, Dory AB, deVilliers AJ, Stocker H, Wigle DT (1985) Lung cancer mortality and radiation exposure among the Newfoundland fuorspar miners. In: Stocker H (ed) Occupational radiation safety in mining. Proceedings of the International Conference. Canadian Nuclear Association, Toronto, pp 354–364

Muller J, Wheeler WC, Gentleman JF, Suranyi G, Kusiak R (1985) Study of mortality of Ontario miners. In: Stocker (ed) Occupational radiation safety in mining. Proceedings of the International Conference. Canadian Nuclear Association, Toronto, pp 335–343

Nero AV, Schwehr MB, Nazaroff WW, Revzan KL (1986) Distribution of airborne radon-222 concentrations in US homes. Science 234: 992–997

NIOSH: National Institute for Occupational Safety and Health (1987) A recommended standard for occupational exposure to radon progeny in underground mines. US Department of Health and Human Services, Washington DC

Passey RD (1962) Some problems of lung cancer. Lancet ii: 107–112

Pershagen G, Damber L, Falk R (1984) Exposure to radon in dwellings and lung cancer: a pilot study. In: Berglund B, Lindvall T, Sundell J (eds) Indoor air. Radon, passive smoking, particulates and housing epidemiology, vol 2. Swedish Council for Building Research, Stockholm, pp 73–78

Placek V, Smid A, Sevc J, Tomasek L, Vernerova P (1983) Late effects at high and very low exposure levels of the radon daughters. In: Broerse JJ, Barendsen GW, Kal HB, Vanderkogel AJ (eds) Radiation research – somatic and genetic effects. Proceedings of 7th International Congress of Radiation Research. Nijhoff, Amsterdam

Radford EP, Renard KG SC (1984) Lung cancer in Swedish iron miners exposed to low doses of radon daughters. N Engl J Med 310: 1485–1494

Samet JM, Kutvirt DM, Waxweiler RJ, Key CR (1984) Uranium mining and lung cancer in Navajo men. N Engl J Med 310: 1481–1484

Schmier H, Wick A (1985) Results from a survey of indoor radon exposures in the Federal Republic of Germany. Sci Total Environ 45: 307–310

Sevc J, Kunz E, Plasek V (1976) Lung cancer in uranium miners and longterm exposure to radon daughter products. Health Phys 30: 433–437

Simpson SG, Comstock GW (1983) Lung cancer and housing characteristics. Arch Environ Health 38: 248–251

Sluis-Cremer GK, Walthers LG, Sichel HF (1967) Chronic bronchitis in miners and nonminers: an epidemiological survey of a community in the goldmining area in Transvaal. Br J Ind Med 24: 1–12

Stranden E (1987) Radon-222 in Norwegian dwellings. In: Hopke PK (ed) Radon and its decay products – occurrence, properties and health effects. American Chemical Society, Washington DC, pp 70–83

Stranden E, Berteig L, Ugletveit F (1979) A study on radon in dwellings. Health Phys 36: 413–421

Svensson C, Eklund G, Pershagen G (1987) Indoor exposure to radon from the ground and bronchial cancer in women. Int Arch Occup Environ Health 59: 123–131

Svensson C, Pershagen G, Klominek J (1988) Lung cancer in women and type of dwelling in relation to radon exposure. In: Svensson C Lung cancer etiology in women. Thesis. Karolinska Institute, Stockholm

Swedjemark GA, Buren A, Mjönes L (1987) Radon levels in Swedish homes: a comparison of the 1980s with the 1950s. In: Hopke PK (ed) Radon and its decay products – occurrence, properties and health effects. American Chemical Society, Washington DC, pp 85–96

Tirmarche M, Brenot J, Piechowski J, Chameaud J, Pradel J (1985) The present state of an epidemiological study of uranium miners in France. In: Stocker H (ed) Occupational Radiation Safety in Mining vol 1. Canadian Nuclear Association, Toronto, pp 344–349

Wagoner JK, Miller RW, Lundin Jr FE, Fraumeni JF, Haij NE (1963) Unusual mortality among a group of underground metal miners. N Engl J Med 269: 281–289

Wald NJ, Idle M, Boreham J, Bailey A (1983) Inhaling and lung cancer: an anomaly explained. Br Med J 287: 1273–1275

Walsh PJ (1970) Radiation dose to the respiratory tract of uranium miners – a review of the literature: Environ Res 3: 14–36

Wang X, Huang X et al. (1984) Radon and miners' lung cancer. Zhonghus Fangshe Yixue yu Fanghu Zazhi 4: 10–14

Waxweiler RJ, Wagoner JK, Archer VE (1973) Mortality of potash workers. J Occup Med 15: 486–489

Waxweiler RJ, Roscoe RJ, Archer VE, Thun MJ, Wagoner JK, Lundin E (1981) Mortality follow-up through 1977 of the white underground uranium miners cohort examined by the United States Public Health Service. In: Gomez M (ed) Radiation hazards in mining: control, measurement and medical aspects. Society of Mining Engineers of the American Institute of Mining, Metallurgical, and Petroleum Engineers, New York, 823–830

WHO (1972) Health hazards of the human environment. World Health Organization, Geneva

Wilkinson GS (1985) Gastric cancer in New Mexico counties with significant deposits of uranium. Arch Environ Health 40: 307–312

Cancer Risks Due to Exposure to Electromagnetic Fields

G. Thériault

McGill University, School of Occupational Health, 1130 Pine Avenue West, Montreal, Quebec H3A 1A3, Canada

The association between exposure to electromagnetic fields (EMF) and human cancer was made the object of several recent reviews (Aldrich and Easterley 1987; Coleman and Beral 1988; Kavet and Banks 1986; Savitz and Callel 1987; Sheik 1986).

In this paper, questions addressed are: (a) the interaction of electric and magnetic fields with the human body; (b) the strength of the evidence of carcinogenicity to humans, and (c) the recent developments in measuring human exposure to extremely low frequency (60 Hz) electric and magnetic fields.

Interaction of Electric and Magnetic Fields with the Human Body

From accidents of electrocution, it is known that the human body is a good conductor of electricity. Under a uniform low intensity electric field, the human body, like any other conducting object, causes a distortion of the electric field (Sheppard and Eisenbud 1977). Electric radiation enters the body at a perpendicular angle. As a consequence, measuring electric field exposure is complex since exposure will change with each movement of the body. In addition, electrical radiation is distorted by the presence of any conductive object in the vicinity of a person. The magnetic field, contrary to the electric field, is not distorted by the human body. It passes directly through buildings and most features in the environment.

Both electric and magnetic fields induce internal currents in the body (Bridges and Preache 1981).

In the case of electric fields, current enters the body at various points and leaves it through the parts that are in contact with the ground. The magnetic field induces a secondary electric current which remains within the body and travels in a circular pattern.

Transmission lines which transport electricity over long distances generate both electric and magnetic fields. The intensity of those fields is proportional to the amount of electricity that circulates in the lines. Electric fields are highest at approximately 20 m from the centre of the line and can reach 10 kV/m for wires

Recent Results in Cancer Research, Vol. 120

that transport 765 kV whereas magnetic fields are highest directly under the line and can reach 250 mG (IERE 1987).

Electric appliances in the home generate electric as well as magnetic fields. Tables 1 and 2 give the intensity of those fields measured at 30 cm from the source.

For electric fields, most appliances will generate fields of intensities varying between 30 and 90 V/m with one major exception, electric blankets which generate the highest field of the order of 250 V/m (Sheppard and Eisenbud 1977). For magnetic fields, the appliances which generate the highest fields are microwave ovens, electric can openers, vacuum cleaners and electric blankets (Gauger 1985).

Occupational environments can expose workers to magnetic field strengths which are 100 to 1000 times higher than household fields (Coleman and Beral 1988).

Assessment of the Evidence of Carcinogenicity to Humans

The possibility that chronic exposure to low intensity EMF may cause cancer in man has only been raised recently. Epidemiological evidence accumulated so far essentially comes from environmental and occupational studies.

Table 1. Typical values of electric fields generated by electric appliances. Based on data given in IERE (1988)

Appliances	Electric field (V/m) at 30 cm from appliance
Incandescent light bulb	2
Electric cooking	4
Vacuum cleaner	16
Color TV	30
Coffee pot	30
Vaporizer	40
Toaster	40
Hair dryer	40
Hand mixer	50
Iron	60
Refrigerator	60
Stereo sound equipment	90
Broiler	130
Electric blanket	250

Table 2. Typical values of magnetic fields generated by electric appliances. Based on data given in IERE (1988)

Appliances	Range of measured fields (mG)
Electric ranges	3–50
Ovens	1–50
Microwaves	40–90
Garbage disposals	8–12
Dishwashers	7–14
Refrigerators	< 0.1–3
Washers	2–20
Dryers	0.7–3
Coffee makers	0.7–1.5
Toasters	0.6–8
Crock pots	0.8–1.5
Irons	1–4
Can openers	30–300
Mixers	6–150
Blenders	5–25
Vacuum cleaners	20–200
Portable heaters	1.5–40
Fans	0.2–40
Hair dryers	< 1–100
Shavers	1–100
Televisions	0.3–20
Fluorescent fixtures	20–40
Desk lamps	5–20
Saws	10–300
Drills	25–40

Environmental Studies

Environmental studies first addressed the question of cancer occurrence in children. In 1979 Wertheimer and Leeper observed that children who died of cancer lived in residences where electric and magnetic field exposures were considered higher than residences of controls. Following this observation, Fulton et al. (1980) in Rhode Island and Myers et al. (1985) in the United

Kingdom, were unable to replicate these results whereas Tomenius (1986) in Sweden and Savitz (1987) in the United States, did observe the same association. The most revealing findings of these five case-control studies relate to three health issues: all childhood tumors, childhood leukemia, and central nervous system tumors. With respect to all childhood tumors, clear excesses were observed by Wertheimer and Leeper (1979) and Tomenius (1986), no excess was seen by Myers et al. (1985) whereas Savitz (1987) observed an excess only when wire configuration was used as a measure of exposure in a manner similar to that of Wertheimer.

For childhood leukemia, the evidence of an excess is far less convincing. Except for Wertheimer and Leeper (1979), and to a limited degree Savitz (1987), other authors have failed to show an excess of childhood leukemia associated with exposure to magnetic fields. Three studies have looked at the association between magnetic fields and central nervous system tumors in children (Ahlbom et al. 1987). An excess has been observed by Tomenius (1986) and Wertheimer and Leeper (1979) but not by Savitz (1987).

Other studies have attempted to provide additional information by either looking at cancer in exposed cohorts or by investigating other health issues in relation to EMF exposure. Two cohort studies have been carried out. In the first McDowall (1986) identified through the 1971 census, 8000 persons who lived in houses located near electric transmission facilities, and followed the mortality of the cohort up to 1983. Except for an excess of lung cancer mortality in women, no other positive findings were observed.

Knowing that the highest exposure to electric fields results from sleeping under electric blankets or on waterbeds, Wertheimer and Leeper (1986) investigated a cohort of 673 births among people who had been using these electric devices over a period of 8 years. The study aimed to address the question of the effect of EMF exposure on the fetus or on abortion rates. The authors observed a seasonal pattern in fetal growth and abortion rates in families using electrically heated beds which correlated with the months of the years they were used. Gestation periods were generally longer in users of electrically heated beds for infants conceived in the season where the need for electric bed heating was greatest. Similarly, an excess of reported abortions occurred in the winter months, especially in those months when the mean temperature was coldest.

Perry et al. (1981) selected 598 suicide deaths which occurred between 1969 and 1976 and matched each of them with a random control. Magnetic field intensity was measured at addresses of cases and controls. It was observed that more cases than controls had been exposed to high magnetic fields and that the intensity of the fields was higher among cases.

Wertheimer and Leeper (1982) matched 1179 adult cancers diagnosed between 1967 and 1975 with 1179 controls selected in several ways. Exposure was assessed by looking at wiring configurations around the houses of cases and controls. The following findings were noted: cases were more exposed than controls; there was a dose-response relationship between exposure and cancer; the risk was more pronounced among people under 55 years of age; the main cancers in excess were those of the central nervous system, uterus, and breast, as well as malignant lymphomas, and all cancers.

Finally, Aldrich et al. (1984) reported a cluster of five children who developed an endodermal sinus tumor between 1974 and 1978. They all lived in the same district and all had a high estimated exposure to EMF. The author mentioned that the association with EMF was purely hypothetical and that these children had also been exposed to environmental lead and polycyclic hydrocarbons.

The information gained through the results of the above environmental studies can be summarized as follows:

1. The type of childhood cancer that has been associated with an excess exposure to electromagnetic fields are all cancers (three studies out of four), central nervous system tumors (two studies out of three), and leukemia (two studies out of five).
2. With regard to excesses of adult cancers resulting from exposure to EMF, the findings are contradictory, one study reporting a positive association (Wertheimer and Leeper (1982), and the other negative findings (McDowall 1986). However, the latter study did not have enough power to exclude a two to threefold increased risk.
3. One study found an association between EMF exposure and suicide, but it was not replicated.
4. The effect of electric blankets and waterbeds on pregnancy outcomes are difficult to interpret.
5. The measure of exposure to EMF that was associated with cancer was wire configuration around houses; actual and estimated measurements were less well correlated with excesses of cancer.

Occupational Studies

Several studies have examined the potential cancer risk of EMF exposures in occupational groups. These studies may be classified under three headings: (a) leukemia in electrical workers, (b) leukemia in other workers exposed to EMF, (c) health studies of electrical workers.

Leukemia in Electrical Workers

A series of short papers originating from several countries and gathering information from several sources, have been published between 1982 and 1988 (Calle and Savitz 1985; Coleman et al. 1983; Howe and Lindsay 1983; McDowall 1983; Milham 1982, 1985a, b, 1988; Pearce et al. 1985; Wright et al. 1982). The great majority of these studies have observed an excess of all leukemias among electrical workers, although in many instances, this excess did not reach statistical significance. Most statistical analyses used in these studies were proportional risk ratios.

Leukemia in Other Workers Exposed to EMF

Five comprehensive mortality studies of aluminum workers have been published (Andersen et al. 1982; Gibbs 1985; Milham 1979; Mur et al. 1987; Rockette and Vincent 1983). Although significant excess of acute leukemia, lymphosarcoma, and reticulum cell sarcoma were observed in only one study (Milham 1979), it is remarkable that most standardized mortality ratios (SMRs) were over 100. This is rather worrisome considering that the overall mortality of these workers, taking into consideration the healthy worker effect, gives an SMR for all causes of about 80.

Two recent case-control within cohort studies have led to unexpected findings. Underground coal miners represent an occupational group exposed to EMF. High voltage overhead power distribution lines are common in mines and converters in stepdown transformers are used to provide power to mining equipment. Gilman et al. (1985) examined the risk to coal miners of exposure to EMF in a case-control study of 40 leukemia cases and 160 controls who died of causes other than cancer. A statistically significant risk for all leukemias, chronic lymphocytic leukemia, and myelogenous leukemia was observed for workers with 24 or more years of underground mining.

Similarly, in a matched case-control study conducted in naval shipyard workers with the intent of studying the relationship between exposure to ionizing radiation and leukemia, Stern et al. (1986), observed that leukemia was associated not with ionizing radiation but with occupation such as done by electricians and welders, occupations known to have high exposures to EMF.

Other Studies of Electrical Workers

In a search for stronger evidence of leukemia associated with occupational exposure to EMF, six cohort studies have been conducted in the following occupational groups: electrical workers, electronic and electrical manufacturing industry workers, telecommunications workers, electrical engineers, powerlinemen, and power station operators (Olin et al. 1985; Swerdlow 1983; Tornqvist et al. 1986; Vagero and Olin 1983; Vagero et al. 1985; Wertheimer and Leeper 1982). Sample sizes were reasonably large and observation periods extended over 30 years. Surprisingly, no excesses of leukemia were observed, but excess of cancers of the pharynx, lung, and skin melanomas were noted.

Four case-control studies of central nervous system cancers have been conducted in occupational settings. In comparing the occupational history and exposure to EMF, based on panel rating, between 951 cases of brain cancer deaths and 951 randomly selected controls dying of noncancer causes, Lin et al. (1985) observed elevated odds ratios for electricians, electric and electronic engineers, and utility workers. He also reported a dose-response relationship between the risk of brain cancer and exposure to EMF. Thomas et al. (1987) compared the occupational history of 435 cases of brain cancer deaths with that of 386 nonbrain cancer deaths and reported elevated odds ratios for workers exposed to microwave-radio-frequency radiation and the manufacture and repair of electronic equipment, as well as for electric-electronic workers. In a population-based case-control study of 202 males who died from gliomas in 1969–1978, Speers et al. (1988) observed a dose-related increased risk for brain cancer among male workers employed in occupations associated with electric or electromagnetic fields. Finally, excess deaths from neuroblastoma have been noted in children whose fathers were exposed to EMF (Spitz and Johnson 1985).

Results from these occupational studies allow the following conclusions to be drawn:

1. The combined results of the studies of electrical workers show a relative risk of 1.18 (confidence interval 1.09–1.29) for all leukemias and a relative risk of 1.46 (confidence interval 1.27–1.65) for acute myeloid leukemia (Coleman et al. 1983).
2. The excesses of leukemia observed in mortality studies conducted from mortality or cancer registries are poorly corroborated by cohort studies.
3. From cohort studies, the type of adult cancers associated with exposure to EMF are: all cancers (three studies out of six), skin melanoma (three studies out of six), non-Hodgkin's lymphoma, lung cancer, and pharyngeal cancer (one study out of five for each tumor type).
4. Elevated odds ratios for brain cancer have been reported in four case-control studies.

Assessment of Overall Causality

The classical criteria for causality may be applied to assess the evidence accumulated thus far. The consistency of the results is not obvious. Although similar observations in occupational groups have been published from different countries using different sources of information, one must realize that from one study to another, the cancer type in excess is not always the same and the occupation in which this excess is observed varies greatly from one study to another.

The strength of the association is moderate to weak. Among exposed workers, the risk can be estimated at 1.18 for all leukemias and at 1.46 for acute myeloid leukemia. For cancer in children, the association is only suggestive. In terms of specificity of the disease, three cancer types have been most commonly observed: acute myeloid leukemia, brain cancer, and skin melanoma.

Most of the reported studies are plagued with several weaknesses: the sample size is often small; many analyses are based on proportional mortality or incidence ratios; exposure to electromagnetic fields has been assessed indirectly without precise measurements, often being based only on occupational titles and classifications; confounding factors have never been considered.

The biological plausibility of an association between cancer and EMF has long been the object of debate. There has been an important breakthrough recently, particularly with regard to cell membrane windowing and ACTH-mediated effects which suggests that exposure to low level 60 Hz EMF may interfere with cellular and hormonal mechanisms in biological tissues (Aldrich and Easterley 1987). It is to be expected that more research on the mechanisms by which EMF can interfere with biological material will be forthcoming.

Measurement of Exposure

One of the major limitations of the human studies reviewed is the quantitative assessment of exposure. The excess risk observed, be it in electrical workers or in children living in residences located in the vicinity of transmission lines means little unless one can demonstrate that these subjects had a higher exposure than people considered not exposed. To assess exposures, several means have been imagined, most of them indirect measurements. One approach has been to observe the electrical wiring configuration around houses. This estimate of exposure assessment was first used by Wertheimer et al. (Wertheimer and Leeper 1979) and has been utilized by other authors afterward. Based on the size of the wires, the closeness of the house to these wires, and the distance to transformers and power stations, investigators have been able to classify homes into groups considered as having high, medium, or low current configurations. Although indirect, this means of assessment has turned out to be reasonably accurate for magnetic fields but less so for electric fields (Kaune et al. 1987).

Another way to assess exposure has been to perform spot measurements near the front doors of houses and over or under electrical wires, to calculate an estimated exposure for people living in the houses. Other authors have based their research design on residences built alongside electrical lines or in the vicinity of electrical power stations.

In most recent studies, actual measurements of electric and magnetic fields have been carried out at the time of interview in rooms where cases and controls lived. Measurements have been made with all the appliances turned on and off to obtain an overall estimate of exposure.

Finally, most occupational studies have simply been based on the occupational history of the workers and on job description and classification. This is particularly troublesome because occupations do not necessarily mean higher exposure, and occupational groups may turn out to be made of heterogeneous exposure.

Dosimetry

All measurements done so far have been instantaneous spot measurements, with no continuous monitoring, the reason being that instruments to carry out continuous monitoring did not exist. Such instruments, however, have been

Table 3. Comparison of work, nonwork, sleeping, and overall weekly time-weighted average (TWA) exposures for utility workers (occupationally exposed to EMF) and nonutility workers (exposed to background EMF)

	60 Hz electric fields							
	Work		Nonwork		Sleep[b]		Weekly TWA	
Group	Geometric mean (V/m)	95% CI[a]	Geometric mean (V/m)	95% CI	Geometric mean (V/m)	95% CI	Geometric mean (V/m)	95% CI
Exposed	37.0	(20.0–67.6)	10.9	(8.5–13.6)	10.6	(6.9–14.5)	21.5	(15.1–30.7)
Background	4.9	(3.6–6.6)	10.7	(7.2–15.3)	19.0	(10.5–34.7)	13.7	(8.9–21.0)
Ratio:								
exposed/background	7.6***	(3.9–14.9)	1.0	(0.7–1.6)	0.6	(0.3–1.1)	1.6	(0.9–2.7)

	60 Hz magnetic fields							
	Work		Nonwork		Sleep		Overall weekly TWA	
Group	Geometric mean (μT)	95% CI	Geometric mean (μT)	95% CI	Geometric mean (μT)	95% CI	Geometric mean (μT)	95% CI
Exposed	1.31	(0.91–1.87)	0.31	(0.22–0.45)	0.16	(0.10–0.26)	0.50	(0.40–0.63)
Background	0.16	(0.13–0.21)	0.19	(0.15–0.24)	0.14	(0.09–0.21)	0.17	(0.13–0.22)
Ratio:								
exposed/background	8.1***	(5.5–12.1)	1.6*	(1.1–2.5)	1.2	(0.6–2.2)	2.9***	(2.1–4.0)

	5–20 MHz transient electromagnetic fields							
	Work		Nonwork		Sleep		Overall weekly TWA	
Group	Geometric mean (ppm)	95% CI	Geometric mean (ppm)	95% CI	Geometric mean (ppm)	95% CI	Geometric mean (ppm)	95% CI
Exposed	0.126	(0.040–0.427)	0.013	(0.004–0.078)	0.002	(< 0.001–0.006)	0.042	(0.20–0.138)
Background	0.002	(0.001–0.005)	0.002	(0.001–0.006)	0.001	(< 0.001–0.001)	0.002	(0.001–0.005)
Ratio:								
exposed/background	65.0***	(15.8–263.0)	9.0**	(1.9–20.4)	1.5	(0.6–4.1)	17.0***	(7.2–89.1)

Significance of difference between exposed and background groups (two-sided *t*-test): $P < 0.001$ – ***; $P < 0.01$ – **; $P < 0.05$ – *.

[a] 95% Confidence interval on mean exposures.

[b] Dosimeter not worn; field measured near the bed.

designed recently and I would like to report on results that we have obtained in a group of utility workers in the province of Quebec.

The dosimeter is a pocket-sized battery-operated device measuring magnetic fields, electric fields, and combined electromagnetic fields called transients every minute during 14 days (Deadman et al. 1988). The dosimeter has a memory, and at the end of 14 days, it is read by a computer, and the profile of the exposure is displayed on the screen.

Levels of exposure may be displayed by day of the week or by hours of the day. In this way, exposure during work hours can be differentiated from exposure in the evening, at night, or over the weekend. Simultaneously, exposure can be expressed as a histogram giving the distribution of the frequency of several exposures over the selected time period.

We have tried to determine if utility workers have higher exposure than nonutility workers and if there are differences of exposure between occupations within the utility workforce. Exposure is read separately for the work, nonwork, and sleeping hours for each day of the week. The geometric mean of each of these exposures is used as a summary assessment as well as to compute a weekly time-weighted average.

So far, measurements have been carried out on 27 utility workers occupationally exposed to EMF and on 16 nonutility workers considered to be exposed to background EMF. As shown in Table 3, during working hours, the mean geometric magnetic field exposure of exposed workers was 1.31 microteslas (μT) whereas for the background group it was 0.16 μT for a ratio exposed to background of 8.1 which is statistically different. During nonworking hours which correspond to activities in the evening and off work, there still was a difference between the exposed group and the background group with a ratio exposed to background of 1.6. During sleeping hours, there was no difference between the two groups. The overall weekly time-weighted average showed a ratio exposed to background of 2.9 which is significant although less remarkable than the ratio observed during working hours, reflecting a dilution of exposure through the addition of nonworking hours. Similar results have been obtained for electric field exposures. With regard to transient exposures, which corresponds to exposure to fields of very high intensity, the difference between the exposed and nonexposed group was much larger with a ratio of 65 for working hours and 17 for the overall weekly time-weighted average.

To investigate exposures in occupations within utility works, measurements were carried out for several occupational groups. Table 4 illustrates the results obtained. Important differences between occupations within the utility industry are noted. Concerning electric fields, transmission linemen have the highest exposure, followed by distribution linemen and apparatus electricians. With regard to magnetic fields, splicers have the highest exposure. As for transient electromagnetic fields, it is the generating station operator that has the highest exposure followed by transmission linemen and distribution linemen.

The number of samples carried out so far is small and these findings can only be indicative. Nevertheless, they show that differences of exposure exist between individuals and occupations. The availability of the dosimeter opens a new field

Table 4. Mean weekly exposures during work for occupations within electric utility works

Occupation	Individuals (n)	E-field (V/m)		B-field (μT)		HFT-field (ppm)	
		Geometric mean	95% CI	Geometric mean		Geometric mean	
Lineman (distribution)	10	62.5	(34.7–112.2)	1.453	(0.776–2.754)	0.286	(0.024–3.162)
Apparatus electrician (transmission)	10	34.9	(11.0–112.2)	1.134	(0.550–2.344)	0.012	(0.001–0.115)
Lineman (transmission)	2	418.9	–	1.313	–	3.051	–
Splicer (distribution)	2	6.7	–	2.075	–	0.038	–
Apparatus mechanics	2	4.7	–	1.175	–	0.044	–
Generating station assistant operator	1	5.0	–	1.136	–	7.965	–
All exposed occupations	27	37.0	(20.0–67.6)	1.306	(0.914–1.866)	0.129	(0.040–0.427)
Background group	16	4.9	(3.6–6.6)	0.161	(0.126–0.205)	0.002	(0.001–0.004)

E-field, electric field (volt per meter); B-field, magnetic field (microtesla); HFT-field, high frequency transient electric field (parts per million)

of research to test the hypothesis of a relationship between EMF and cancer in environmental as well as in occupational settings.

References

Ahlbom A, Albert EN, Fraser-Smith AC, Grodzinsky AJ, Marron MT, Martin AP, Persingter MA, Shelanski ML, Wolpow ER (1987) Biological effects of power line fields. New York State power lines project. Scientific Advisory Panel Final Report.

Aldrich TE, Easterley CE (1987) Electromagnetic fields and public health. Environ Health Perspect 75: 159–171

Aldrich TE, Clorieux A, Castro S (1984) Florida cluster of five children with endodermal sinus tumors. Oncology 41: 233–238

Andersen A, Dahlberg BE, Magnus K, Wannag A (1982) Risk of cancer in the Norwegian aluminum industry. 29: 295–298

Bridges JE, Preache M (1981) Proc IEEE 69: 1092

Calle E, Savitz DA (1985) Leukaemia in occupational groups with presumed exposure to electrical and magnetic fields. N Engl J Med 313: 1476–1477

Coleman M, Beral V (1988) A review of epidemiological studies of the health effects of living near or working with electricity generation and transmission equipment. Int J Epidemiol 17: 1–13

Coleman M, Bell J, Skeet R (1983) Leukaemia incidence in electrical workers. Lancet i: 982–983

Deadman JE, Camus M, Armstrong BG et al. (1988) Occupational and residential 60 Hz electromagnetic fields and high frequency electric transients: exposure assessment using a new dosimeter. Am Ind Hyg Assoc J 49(8): 409–419

Fulton JP, Cobb S, Preble L, Leone L, Forman E (1980) Electrical wiring configuration and childhood leukemia in Rhode Island. Am J Epidemiol 111: 292–296

Gauger JR (1985) Household appliance magnetic field survey. IEEE Trans PAS-104, no 9

Gibbs GW (1985) Mortality of aluminum reduction plant workers, 1950 through 1977. J Occup Med 27: 761–770

Gilman PA, Ames RG, McCawley A (1985) Leukemia risk among U.S. white male coal miners. J Occup Med 27: 669–671

Howe GR, Lindsay JP (1983) A follow-up study of a ten-percent sample of the Canadian Labour Force. 1. Cancer mortality in males. 1965–73. J NCI 70: 37–44

IERE: International Electric Research Exchange (1988) Epidemiological studies relating human health to electric and magnetic fields: criteria for evaluation. Final report, Palo Alto, June 22, 1988

Kaune WT, Stevens RG, Callahan NJ et al. (1987) Residential magnetic and electric fields. Bioelectromagnetics 8: 315–335

Kavet RI, Banks RS (1986) Emerging issues in extremely-low-frequency electric and magnetic field health research. Environ Res 39: 386–404

Lin RS, Dischinger PC, Conde J, Farrell KP (1985) Occupational exposure to electromagnetic fields and the occurrence of brain tumours: an analysis of possible associations. J Occup Med 27: 413–419

McDowall ME (1983) Leukaemia mortality in electrical workers in England and Wales. Lancet i: 246

McDowall ME (1986) Mortality of persons resident in the vicinity of electricity transmission facilities. Br J Cancer 53: 271–279
Milham S (1979) Mortality in aluminum reduction plant workers. J Occup Med 21: 475–480
Milham S (1982) Mortality from leukemia in workers exposed to electrical and magnetic fields. N Engl J Med 307: 249
Milham S (1985a) Silent keys: leukaemia mortality in amateur radio operators. Lancet i: 811
Milham S (1985b) Mortality in workers exposed to electromagnetic fields. Environ Health Perspect 62: 297–300
Milham S (1988) Increased mortality in amateur radio operators due to lymphatic and hematopoietic malignancies. Am J Epidemiol 127: 50–54
Mur JM, Moulin JJ, Meyer-Bisch C, Massin N, Coulon JP, Loulergue J (1987) Mortality of aluminum reduction plant workers in France. Int J Epidemiol 16: 257–264
Myers A, Cartwright RA, Bonnell JA, Male CR, Cartwright SC (1985) Overhead power lines and childhood cancer. In: International Conference on electric and magnetic fields in medicine and biology, London.
Olin R, Vagero D, Ahlbom A (1985) Mortality experience of electrical engineers. Br J Ind Med 42: 211–212
Pearce NE, Sheppart AR, Howard JK, Fraser J, Lilley BM (1985) Leukaemia in electrical workers in New Zealand. Lancet i: 811–812
Perry FS, Reichmanis M, Marino AA, Becker RO (1981) Environmental power frequency magnetic fields and suicide. Health Phys 41: 267–277
Rockette HE, Vincent CA (1983) Mortality studies of aluminum reduction plant workers: potroom and carbon departments. J Occup Med 25: 349–557
Savitz DA (1987) Case-control study of childhood cancer and residential exposure to electric and magnetic fields. Report to the New York State Department of Health, Power Lines Project.
Savitz DA, Calle EE (1987) Leukemia and occupational exposure to electromagnetic fields: review of epidemiologic surveys. J Occup Med 29: 47–51
Sheikh H (1986) Exposure to electromagnetic fields and the risk of leukemia. Arch Environ Health 41: 56–63
Sheppard AR, Eisenbud M (1977) Biological effects of electric and magnetic fields of extremely low frequency. New York University Press, New York
Speers MA, Dobbins JG, Miller VS (1988) Occupational exposures and brain cancer mortality: a preliminary study of East Texas residents. Am J Ind Med 13: 629–638
Spitz MR, Johnson CC (1985) Neuroblastoma and paternal occupation: a case-control analysis. Am J Epidemiol 121: 924–929
Stern FB, Waxweiler RA, Beaumont JJ et al. (1986) A case-control study of leukemia at a naval nuclear shipyard. Am J Epidemiol 123: 980–992
Swerdlow AJ (1983) Epidemiology of eye cancer in adults in England and Wales, 1962–1977. Am J Epidemiol 118: 294–300
Thomas TL, Stolley PD, Sternhagen A et al. (1987) Brain tumor mortality among men with electrical and electronics jobs: a case-control study. J NCI 79: 233–238
Tomenius L (1986) 50-Hz electromagnetic environment and the incidence of childhood tumors in Stockholm county. Bioelectromagnetics 7: 191–207
Tornqvist S, Norell S, Ahlbom A, Knave B (1986) Cancer in the electric power industry. Br J Ind Med 43: 212–213

Vagero D, Olin R (1983) Incidence of cancer in the electronics industry: using the new Swedish Cancer Environment Registry as a screening instrument. Br J Ind Med 40: 188–192

Vagero D, Ahlbom A, Olin R, Sahlsten S (1985) Cancer morbidity among workers in the telecommunications industry. Br J Ind Med 42: 191–195

Wertheimer N, Leeper E (1979) Electrical wiring configurations and childhood cancer. Am J Epidemiol 109: 273–284

Wertheimer N, Leeper E (1982) Adult cancer related to electrical wires near the home. Int J Epidemiol 11: 345–355

Wertheimer N, Leeper E (1986) Possible effects of electric blankets and heated waterbeds on fetal development. Bioelectromagnetics. 7: 13–22

Wright WE, Peters JM, Mack TM (1982) Leukemia in workers exposed to electrical and magnetic fields. Lancet ii: 1160–1164

Human Lung Cancer Risks Due to Complex Organic Mixtures of Combustion Emissions

J.L. Mumford[1], X.Z. He[2], and R.S. Chapman[1]

[1] U.S. Environmental Protection Agency, Research Triangle Park, NC 27711, USA
[2] Institute of Environmental Health and Engineering, 29 Nan Wei Road, Beijing, People's Republic of China

Introduction

Man has long been exploiting his environmental resources, including fossil fuels, biomass, and man-made fuels, for purposes such as cooking, heating, transportation, and industrial production. These activities often result in the production of incomplete combustion products, which are made of very complex mixtures that contain thousands of compounds, both organic and inorganic. The organic constituents from these emissions contain aliphatic hydrocarbons, aromatic hydrocarbons, polycyclic aromatic hydrocarbons (PAHs), substituted PAHs, and other polar compounds. These organic compounds are present in the form of gases (e.g., benzene, formaldehyde) and particulate matter. The condensed organic matter is usually adsorbed onto carbonaceous particles to form soot or onto alumina-silica particles such as coal fly ash particles.

Laboratory studies have shown that combustion emissions often contain classes of organic compounds that induce tumours in experimental animals, for example, PAHs, methylated PAHs, nitro-PAHs, and nitrogen-containing heterocyclic compounds (International Agency for Research on Cancer 1983). The organic extracts of particles from combustion emissions from various sources have shown genotoxic and carcinogenic effects in various bioassay systems. Organic emissions such as from combustion of coal, diesel, kerosene, wood, and tobacco have been shown to induce mutation in bacteria (Mumford and Lewtas 1982; Lewtas 1983; Kamens et al. 1984; Kinouchi et al. 1988). Organic emissions from diesel-powered engine exhaust, coke ovens, roofing tar, and tobacco smoke were also found to cause mutation, DNA damage, and chromosomal effects in mammalian cells (Claxton and Huisingh 1980; Lewtas 1985); and these emissions also have shown tumor initiation activity in a mouse skin tumor assay (Nesnow et al. 1982). Ishinishi et al. (1986) reported that exposure of animals to whole diesel exhaust emissions via inhalation induced lung cancer in a dose-response fashion.

In human studies, tobacco smoke is known for being the predominant cause of lung cancer (International Agency for Research on Cancer 1986; US Department of Health and Human Services 1982; Doll and Peto 1978). Coal com-

Recent Results in Cancer Research, Vol. 120

pathology reports on every newly diagnosed cancer case are submitted to the Registry from every hospital and regional pathology service in the province. Reciprocal agreements have also been established with the three other western Canadian provinces under which B.C. residents diagnosed in these provinces are reported to the BCCR. Ascertainment for most sites is considered to be virtually complete. To exclude duplicates, patients treated at the CCABC cancer centres are cross-indexed with the Registry files. Accurate documentation on primary site and histology is available in about 95% of all incident cases.

General Methodology

A self-administered questionnaire[1] requesting detailed life-time job descriptions, occupation and industry titles, duration and period of work, as well as information on ethnic origin, education, and life-time smoking habits, has been submitted since January 1st, 1983, to all male cancer patients aged 20 years and over ascertained by the BCCR. Questions on life-time consumption of alcoholic beverages, which were initially omitted, were added to the questionnaire during the first year of study. The following information is also obtained on each patient: surname and first name, age, residence address and telephone number, as well as the family physician's name and telephone number. Anatomic site and histology of the primary tumor is obtained from the BCCR. Patients seen at the two cancer centres (about 50% of all newly diagnosed patients each year except for non-melanoma skin cancer) are given the questionnaire at their first visit with an explanatory letter and a self-addressed stamped envelope for return.

For patients ascertained solely by the BCCR, all of the above identifying information, except residence address and telephone number, are directly available from the Cancer Registry pathology reports. The missing information is obtained by contacting the patient's physician before the questionnaire, explanatory letter and return, pre-paid envelope are sent. The 2 months delay from the time pathology reports reach the Registry to the time cases are actually registered in the BCCR is avoided by obtaining copies of these reports on the day they are received at the Registry. This procedure was established to minimize the loss to the study of patients who might die during this interval.

All patient names are checked against the Registry master file to eliminate duplicates. Lists of patients are printed every 2 weeks, and the doctors' offices contacted to obtain address information.

Patients who have not returned the questionnaire within 2 weeks are sent a reminder post-card and are then contacted by telephone at 2-week intervals on two occasions. Failure to return the questionnaires after this prompting is taken as evidence of patient's refusal to participate in the study. In the event of a patient's death, an attempt is made to obtain the information from the spouse

[1] Available upon request.

or closest relative. Each questionnaire received is checked and patients are called to obtain missing information.

The anatomic site and pathology of the primary tumor are coded using the 9th revision of the International Classification of Diseases (WHO 1977). Occupations and industries are coded according to the Canadian Standard Industrial Classification and Standard Occupational Classification respectively (Statistics Canada 1981a,b). It is planned to accrue 1000 cases for each major tumor site. This will enable detection of a minimum odds ratio of 2.2 given a 1% exposure among the controls.

Non-Hodgkin's Lymphoma and Squamous Cell Lung Cancer Patients and Controls

Between January 1st, 1983, and December 1st, 1986, completed questionnaires were received from 367 patients with non-Hodgkin's lymphoma (NHL) and from 715 patients with squamous cell lung cancer (SCLC). For each of these tumor types, two age-matched internal controls were randomly selected. For SCLC, bladder cancer and non-squamous cell lung cancer were excluded from the control group. Controls for NHL were obtained from the same control pool.

Analysis

All usual (main life-time employment) occupations and industries with at least five cases were analyzed.

Odds ratios (ORs) adjusted for the following five-level smoking stratification were calculated by conditional logistic regression using PECAN (Breslow and Day 1980; Storer et al. 1983): never smoker; cigarette pack-years (number of cigarettes smoked per day × number of years smoking) < 25, 25–49, > 50; non-cigarette smoker (pipe, cigars) and unknown. Data for usual occupation and usual industry of employment will be presented as follows: ORs statistically significantly increased; ORs > 1.50, non-statistically significant; ORs statistically significantly low.

Results

From January 1st, 1983, to December 31st, 1986, questionnaires were sent to 17 584 patients ascertained by the BCCR, and 10 995 were returned (overall response rate 62.7%). Reasons for not returning the questionnaire are shown in Table 1. The site distribution of the 10 995 cases and the proportion of questionnaires received for each site are shown in Table 2. Excluding unknown primaries and a number of sites classified under "other" and multiple primaries,

Table 1. Reasons for not returning questionnaires

		Number	Percent
Questionnaires sent	17584		
Questionnaires received	10995 (62.7%)		
Questionnaire not returned despite patient being contacted by telephone		1617	24.5
Unable to contact patient by telephone		1285	19.5
Patient deceased[a]		1356	20.6
Patient refusal		1082	16.4
Patient too ill[a]		936	14.2
Lost to follow-up		187	2.9
Language problem		126	1.9

[a] Next of kin could not be contacted or refused to fill out questionnaire.

the response by site was greater than 60% except for lung cancer and for esophageal, stomach, liver and pancreatic cancers (Table 2). Questionnaires were completed by the patient in 80% of the cases and by another person, generally the spouse, in one-fifth of the cases. To assess response bias, an attempt was made to obtain information on marital status, years of schooling, smoking history and usual occupation on all individuals who were sent a questionnaire during a 2-month period but did not return it. Exhaustive means to contact non-responders were implemented including multiple morning, afternoon and evening telephone calls. If the patient was deceased, data were obtained from the next of kin, the patient's family physician and from hospital records. During the 2-month period, 286 non-responders were identified, for whom the required information was obtained in 229 (80%). For each non-responder, two responders matched on age (within 5-year age strata) and cancer site were randomly selected from our data set. No statistically significant differences were observed except for the proportion of married patients, which was significantly lower for the non-responders (data not shown).

The control sites for NHL and for SCLC cases are shown in Table 3, and the characteristics of cases and controls are presented in Table 4.

For NHL, ORs for usual occupation and industry are shown in Tables 5 and 6 respectively. Statistically significantly increased ORs were observed for both occupation and industry in pulp and paper, and for the fishing and furniture industries. Whereas a number of occupations and industries had non-significantly increased ORs > 1.50, no statistically low ORs were noted.

For SCLC, ORs for usual occupation and industry are shown in Tables 7 and 8 respectively. Statistically significantly increased ORs were observed for carpenters, miners, metal processing and machining occupations and for miscellaneous processing occupations, including clay, glass and stone processing as well as chemical, petroleum and plastic material processing. Significantly low ORs

Table 2. Tumour site distribution of 10995 cases and proportion of questionnaires received for each site

Site	ICD-9	Number	Percent	Questionnaires received (%)[a]
Oral cavity and pharynx	140–149	475	4.3	67.7
Esophagus	150	139	1.3	55.2
Stomach	151	298	2.7	51.8
Colon	153	940	8.6	69.1
Rectum	154	712	6.5	65.7
Liver	155	40	0.4	41.5
Pancreas	157	121	1.1	53.4
Larynx	161	244	2.2	67.7
Lung	162	1686	15.3	55.7
Bone and connective tissue	170–171	93	0.8	63.1
Melanoma	172	501	4.6	73.2
Non-melanoma skin	173	1241	11.3	65.8
Prostate	185	1520	13.8	70.1
Testis	186	174	1.6	67.2
Bladder	188	850	7.7	66.0
Kidney	189	289	2.6	71.4
Brain	191	166	1.5	64.0
Hodgkin's disease	201	89	0.8	72.5
Non-Hodgkin's lymphoma	200, 202	367	3.3	66.0
Multiple myeloma	203	99	0.9	71.0
Leukemia	204, 205 207, 210	179	1.6	65.6
Other sites and multiple primaries	-	591	5.4	56.5
Unknown primaries	199	181	1.7	46.3
Total		10995	100.0	

[a] $\frac{\text{Questionnaire received}}{\text{Questionnaire sent}} \times 100.$

were noted for physicians and health professionals. Particularly noteworthy are the significantly elevated ORs observed in various metal-related industries.

Discussion

The 63% response rate obtained in this study compares favourably with the 57% response rate of the U.S. Third National Cancer Survey Interview aimed, in particular, at searching for occupational cancer risks (Williams et al. 1977). The elevated risk of non-Hodgkin's lymphoma found for pulp and paper workers in this study confirms our previous observation based on a proportional mortality study (Gallagher and Threlfall 1985) and the findings of other

Table 3. Control sites (%) for non-Hodgkin's lymphoma and for squamous cell lung cancer

Control sites	Non-Hodgkin's lymphoma[a]	Lung cancer[b]
Prostate	13.8	20.8
Colon	12.9	15.0
Non-melanoma skin	11.2	12.1
Rectum	10.4	10.3
Melanoma	8.6	3.7
Oral cavity	6.9	5.5
Leukemia	4.6	2.3
Stomach	4.5	4.5
Kidney	4.1	4.3
Other	23.0	21.5

[a] Bladder and all histologic types of lung cancer excluded from the control group.
[b] Bladder and all non-squamous cell lung cancer excluded from the control group.

Table 4. Characteristics of cases and controls

Characteristics	Non-Hodgkin's lymphoma	Controls	Lung cancer	Controls
Number	367	734	715	1430
Caucasian (%)	92.9	95.1	95.5	96.0
Married (%)	85.6	80.8	80.1	83.3
Mean age (years) ± SD	59.8 ± 0.78	59.8 ± 0.55	67.8 ± 0.35	67.8 ± 0.24
Mean years of schooling ± SD	10.5 ± 0.11	10.2 ± 0.08	9.5 ± 0.10	9.8 ± 0.07
University education (%)	38.4	33.0	21.6	26.0
Cigarette smoking				
Ever smoker (%)	80.8	76.5	98.3	91.7
Current smoker (%)	26.7	31.4	35.1	26.3
Mean age starting smoking ± SD	17.8 ± 0.27	17.8 ± 0.21	17.3 ± 0.16	18.3 ± 0.15
Mean age stopping smoking ± SD	46.6 ± 1.02	47.5 ± 0.78	61.2 ± 0.51	50.5 ± 0.49
Mean number of cigarettes smoked ± SD	20.7 ± 0.70	22.0 ± 0.56	25.7 ± 0.52	20.2 ± 0.38
Mean years of smoking cigarettes ± SD	29.3 ± 0.90	31.0 ± 0.68	44.4 ± 0.43	34.4 ± 0.46
Mean pack-years[a] ± SD	31.0 ± 1.41	35.0 ± 1.26	56.9 ± 1.25	36.1 ± 0.82

SD, standard deviation.
[a] Pack-years: number of cigarettes smoked daily × years of cigarette smoking.

Table 5. Non-Hodgkin's lymphoma risk by usual occupation

SOC[a]	Title	Cases (*n*)	Odds ratio	95% CI	*P*
825	Pulp and paper	5	10.0	1.2–85.6	0.009
811; 822–827, 829	Mineral and metal processing	5	1.7	0.5–5.5	0.39
931	Material handling	14	1.7	0.8–3.3	0.16
871	Excavating, grading	7	2.0	0.7–5.7	0.20
711; 718, 719	Farming	17	0.6	0.4–1.1	0.08

[a] Canadian Standard Occupational Classification (Statistics Canada 1981b).
CI, confidence interval.

Table 6. Non-Hodgkin's lymphoma risk by usual industry

SIC[a]	Title	Cases (*n*)	Odds ratio	95% CI	*P*
62	Furniture	5	5.0	1.0, 25.8	0.03
271	Pulp and paper	7	3.5	1.0, 12.0	0.03
06	Mining	9	1.6	0.7, 3.9	0.27
30	Metal fabricating	5	1.7	0.5, 5.5	0.39
40	Building construction	17	1.8	0.9, 3.6	0.09
48	Communication	9	1.7	0.7, 4.5	0.24

[a] Canadian Standard Industrial Classification (Statistics Canada 1981a).

Table 7. Squamous cell lung cancer risk by usual occupation

SOC[a]	Title	Cases (*n*)	Odds ratio	95% CI	*P*
61	Service	79	1.5	1.0, 2.1	0.029
77	Mining	20	2.2	1.1, 4.3	0.026
811; 813, 814	Mineral and metal processing	16	19.8	4.0, 98.3	0.001
815–817	Miscellaneous processing	6	12.8	1.8, 90.9	0.005
831, 833	Metal machining	35	2.1	1.2, 3.6	0.010
878	Carpenter	24	2.5	1.3, 4.9	0.006
718, 719	Farm workers	19	1.7	1.0, 3.0	0.11
821, 822	Food processing	18	1.7	0.8, 3.6	0.17
911	Air transport	7	2.1	0.7, 6.1	0.19
31	Medicine/health	8	0.4	0.2, 0.9	0.025
51	Sales	55	0.6	0.4, 0.9	0.006

[a] Candian Standard Occupational Classification (Statistics Canada 1981b).

Table 8. Squamous cell lung cancer risk by usual industry

SIC[a]	Title	Cases (*n*)	Odds ratio	95% CI	*P*
29	Primary metal	18	3.8	1.6, 9.0	0.002
30	Metal fabricating	15	2.8	1.1, 6.9	0.025
97	Personal services	9	2.8	1.0, 7.9	0.044
061	Metal mining	20	3.1	1.5, 6.4	0.002
06	Mining	22	1.8	1.0, 3.3	0.059
36	Petroleum	7	4.1	0.9, 20.0	0.068
91	Accommodation	11	1.7	0.7, 4.2	0.29
92	Food and beverage	13	1.6	0.7, 3.8	0.29

[a] Canadian Standard Industrial Classification (Statistics Canada 1981a).

investigators (Hardell 1979). However, the excess non-Hodgkin's lymphoma risk previously documented in United States farmers. (Blair et al. 1985; Cantor 1981; Hoar et al. 1986) was not observed, possibly due to differences in exposure levels or in the type of herbicide and pesticide use.

Although cigarette smoking is the single major cause of bronchogenic carcinoma, a number of lung carcinogens have been identified in the workplace, and several occupations and industrial processes have been found to be associated with an increased lung cancer risk (Merletti and Segnan 1988). The elevated ORs particularly noted for SCLC in our study for occupations and industries involving exposures to minerals and metals confirm the results of our previous occupational mortality study in British Columbia (Gallagher and Threlfall 1983), as well as the observations of other investigators (Kvale et al. 1986).

Hypothesis-generating studies derived from large data-bases have a number of limitations. Due to the number of comparisons made, associations which appear significant may arise due to chance. On the other hand, for occupations and industries with small numbers of cases, the power to detect an excess risk may be low. In this study, wide confidence intervals were observed for several occupation and industry groups with small numbers. However, the fact that the main results of this analysis, namely an increased risk of NHL for pulp and paper workers and of SCLC for metal workers, confirm those of a population-based mortality study in British Columbia strongly suggests that these findings are not due to chance. A final analysis of SCLC will be undertaken when the planned accrual of 1000 cases is completed.

References

Blair A, Malker H, Cantor KP, Burmeister L, Wilkund K (1985) Cancer among farmers: a review. Scand J Work Environ Health 11: 397–407

Breslow NE, Day NE (1980) Statistical methods in cancer research, Vol. 1. The analysis of case-control studies (International Agency for Research on Cancer, Lyon.) (IARC scientific publ no. 32)

Cantor KD (1981) Farming and mortality from non-Hodgkin's lymphoma: a case-control study. Int J Cancer 29: 239–247

Gallagher RP, Threlfall WJ (1983) Cancer mortality in metal workers. Can Med Assoc J 129: 1191–1194

Gallagher RP, Threlfall WJ (1985) Cancer risk in wood and pulp workers. In: Stich H (ed) Carcinogens and mutagens in the Environment, vol 5. CRC, Boca Raton Fl, pp 125–137

Hardell L (1979) Malignant lymphoma of histiocytic type and exposure to phenoxyacetic acids or chlorophenols. Lancet i: 55–56

Hoar SK, Blair A, Holmes FF, Boysen CD, Robel RJ, Hoover R, Fraumeni JF Jr (1986) Agricultural herbicide use and risk of lymphoma and soft-tissue sarcoma. JAMA 256: 1141–1147

Jarvisalo J, Tola S, Korkala M-L, Jarvinen E (1984) A cancer register-based case study of occupations of patients with acute myeloid leukemia. Cancer 54: 785–790

Kvale G, Bjelke E, Hench I (1986) Occupational exposure and lung cancer risk. Int J Cancer 37: 185–193

McCrea Curnen MG, Thompson WD, Heston JF, Flannery JT (1984) Cancer prevention: the tumor registry connection. Cancer Detect Prev 7: 191–199

McLaughlin JK, Malker HSR, Malker BK, Stone BJ, Ericsson JLE, Blot WJ, Weiner JA, Fraumeni JF Jr (1987) Registry-based analysis of occupational risks for primary liver cancer in Sweden. Cancer Res 47: 287–291

Merletti F, Segnan N (1988) Occupational cancers. In: Silverman AJ, Allwright SPA (eds) Elimination or reduction of diseases? Opportunities for Health Service Action in Europe. Oxford University Press, Oxford, pp 157–177

Pearce NE, Sheppard RA, Keir-Howard J, Fraser J, Lilley BM (1986a) Leukemia among New Zealand agricultural workers. Am J Epidemiol 124: 402–409

Pearce NE, Smith AH, Howard JK, Sheppard RA, Giles HJ, Teague CA (1986b) Case-control study of multiple myeloma and farming. Br J Cancer 54: 493–500

Statistics Canada (1981a) Standard industrial classification 1980. Statistics Canada, Ottawa (catalogue 12–501E; ISBN 0–660–10672–8)

Statistics Canada (1981b) Standard Occupational Classification 1980. Statistics Canada, Ottawa, (catalogue 12–565E; ISBN 0–660–10673–6)

Storer BE, Wacholder S, Breslow NE (1983) Maximum likelihood fitting of general risk models to stratified data. Appl Stat 32: 177–181

Williams RR, Stegens NL, Goldsmith JR (1977) Associations of cancer site and type with occupation and industry from the third National Cancer Survey Interview. J NCI 59: 1147–1185

WHO: World Health Organization (1977) International classification of diseases, 9th revision. WHO, Geneva

Subject Index

MIX
Papier aus verantwortungsvollen Quellen
Paper from responsible sources
FSC® C105338

If you have any concerns about our products,
you can contact us on
ProductSafety@springernature.com

In case Publisher is established outside the EU,
the EU authorized representative is:
Springer Nature Customer Service Center GmbH
Europaplatz 3, 69115 Heidelberg, Germany

Printed by Libri Plureos GmbH
in Hamburg, Germany